QIGONG FOR TREATING COMMON AILMENTS

QIGONG FOR TREATING COMMON AILMENTS

The Essential Guide to Self-Healing

XU XIANGCAI

YMAA Publication Center
Boston, Mass. USA

YMAA Publication Center
Main Office:
    PO Box 480
    Wolfeboro, NH 03894
    1-800-669-8892 • info@ymaa.com • www.ymaa.com

POD 0913

ISBN-13: 978-1-886969-70-4   ISBN-10: 1-886969-70-1

Edited by David Shapiro
Cover design by Richard Rossiter

Publisher's Cataloging in Publication
(Prepared by Quality Books Inc.)

Xiangcai, Xu
        Qigong for treating common ailments : the
    essential guide to self-healing / by Xu Xiangcai.
    — 2nd ed.
            p. cm — (Practical TCM)
        Includes index.
        LCCN: 00-101607
        ISBN: 1-886969-70-1

        1. Chi k'ung. 2. Alternative medicine.
    I. Title.

            RA781.8.X53 2000   613.7'1
                                QBI00-518

Disclaimer:
The authors and publisher of this material are NOT RESPONSIBLE in any
manner whatsoever for any injury which may occur through reading or following
the instructions in this manual.
The activities, physical or otherwise, described in this material may be too
strenuous or dangerous for some people, and the reader(s) should consult a
physician before engaging in them.

Printed in USA

Editor's Note

Qigong is, in many ways, the most important aspect of Chinese medicine. It contains the information necessary for people to improve their own health without the assistance of doctors. Although it has been practiced in the United States for many years, it has suffered from misunderstanding and, like many aspects of Chinese medicine, it has been unnecessarily shrouded in mystique. Further complicating Qigong practice are the many variations that are available for study and its association with paranormal abilities. Although it provides many of the same benefits as Yoga, Qigong students are often unable to achieve the same level of health as Yoga students because of the lack of clarity surrounding its practice.

As soon as I read the first translation of this book, I knew that it could improve all forms of Qigong practice and open this important field of study to anyone with a sincere interest. All dogmatic and complicated techniques are discarded for clarity. The essence of Qigong is clearly described making it is possible to successfully practice Qigong through careful study. Like many skill based disciplines, Qigong improves in accordance with the time that is given and there are practitioners who do achieve astounding abilities through long-term practice. For most people, however, there is no need to become Qigong masters. There are many benefits to be gained from the most basic aspects of Qigong theory and practice.

Qigong for Treating Common Ailments covers two categories of Qigong therapy, self-directed and outgoing. The former refers to Qigong exercises practiced by patients to keep themselves fit or to cure their own illness. The latter refers to the ability of Qigong masters to treat patients by emitting Qi. This book is organized into five parts: An Introduction to Medical Qigong, The Three Kinds of Qigong Regulation, Various Qigong Exercises, Outgoing Qigong, and Treatment of Illness with Qigong. It is written as a reference for health care professionals and Qigong practitioners and is also intended as a guide for people who practice Qigong for themselves.

This book is carefully constructed and develops from fundamentals to the treatment of disease. Each section provides the foundation for the one that follows. It is best to read the entire book straight through, to get a feel for its structure, and then slowly and carefully begin again, paying close attention to its many details. It has been our goal with this book to clarify each section to the point where independent study is possible. One of the fundamental lessons of Qigong is that the human body is a microcosm of the universe. Over time, Qigong leads to a direct perception of the physical world allowing students to learn on their own. Once this happens its practice becomes easier and more clear, not more complicated. This book will help clarify Qigong theory and practice to anyone involved in its practice and will allow novices to avoid mistakes. Just like Qigong practice, this book reveals itself only though effort. Keep an open mind and remember to avoid complications. Enjoy and good luck.

David Shapiro L. Ac.

Contents

Chapter 4 Emitting Outgoing Qi

Static Exercise for Training Qi • Dynamic Exercise for Training Qi • Double-Nine Yang Exercise • Exercise of Kneading the Abdomen to Strengthen the Active Substance in the Body
Standing Vibrating with Palms Closed to Guide Qi • Single-finger Meditation to Guide Qi • Palm-pushing and Palm-pulling to Guide Qi • Making Three Points Linear to Guide Qi • Making Three Points Circular to Guide Qi • Jumping to Guide Qi in Bursts • Guiding Qi in Fixed Form • Guiding Qi Spirally • Cold and Heat Guidance of Qi
Hand Gestures for Emitting Qi • Hand Manipulations in Emitting Qi • Manipulations with the Hand Touching the Area Being Treated • Manipulations with the Hand off the Area Being Treated • Auxiliary Manipulations • The Forms of Qi Emission • The Sensation of Qi • The Effects of Qi in Patients • The Closing Form of Qi Emission

Chapter 5 Treatment

Deranged Flow of Qi • Stagnation of Qi and Stasis of Blood • Leaking of Genuine (Vital) Qi • Mental Derangement • Management of Temporary Symptoms Emerging during Qigong Exercise

Foreword
By Prof. Dr. Hu Ximing

I am delighted to learn that *Qigong for Treating Common Ailments* will soon come into the world.

Traditional Chinese Medicine (TCM) has experienced many vicissitudes of times but has remained evergreen. It has made great contributions not only to the power and prosperity of our Chinese nation, but also to the enrichment and improvement of world medicine. Unfortunately, differences in nations, states, and languages have slowed down its introduction and continued interest by cultures and nations outside of China. At present, however, an upsurge in learning, researching and applying Traditional Chinese Medicine is unfolding.

In order to maximize the effect of this upsurge and to lead TCM— one of the brilliant cultural heritages of the Chinese nation—to the world, Mr. Xu Xiangcai called forth intellectuals of noble aspirations from Shandong and many other provinces in China. Together, they took charge of the work of both compilation and translation of *Qigong for Treating Common Ailments* in order for TCM to expand and bring benefit to the people of all nations.

With great pleasure, the medical staff both at home and abroad will hail the appearance of this encyclopedia.

I believe that the day when the world's medicine is fully developed will be the day when TCM has spread throughout the world.

I am pleased to give it my recommendation.

Prof. Dr. Hu Ximing

Deputy Minister of the Ministry of Public Health of the People's Republic of China, Director General of the State Administrative Bureau of Traditional Chinese, Medicine and Pharmacology, President of the World Federation of Acupuncture Moxibustion Societies, Member of China Association of Science & Technology, Deputy President of All-China Association of Traditional Chinese Medicine, President of China Acupuncture & Moxibustion Society

Foreword

Mr. Zhang Qiwen

The Chinese nation has been through a long, arduous course of struggling against diseases and has developed its own traditional medicine, Traditional Chinese Medicine and Pharmacology (TCMP). TCMP is a unique, comprehensive, scientific system including both theories and clinical practice.

Some thousand years since its beginnings, TCMP has not only been well preserved, but also continuously developed. It has special advantages, such as remarkable curative effects and few side effects. It is an effective means by which people prevent and treat diseases and keep themselves strong and healthy.

All achievements attained by any nation in the development of medicine are the public wealth of all mankind. They should not be confined within a single country. What is more, the need to set them free to flow throughout the world as quickly and precisely as possible is greater than that of any other kind of science.

During my more than thirty years of being engaged in Traditional Chinese Medicine (TCM), I have been looking forward to the day when TCMP will have spread all over the world and made its contributions to the elimination of diseases of all mankind. However, it is to be deeply regretted that the pace that TCMP is extending outside China has been unsatisfactorily slow due to the major difficulties in expressing its concepts in foreign languages.

Mr. Xu Xiangcai, a teacher of Shandong College of TCM, has sponsored and taken charge of the work of compilation and translation of The English-Chinese of Practical Traditional Chinese Medicine, an extensive series. This work is a great project, a large-scale scientific research, a courageous effort, and a novel creation. I deeply esteem Mr. Xu Xiangcai and his compilers and translators—who have been working day and night for such a long time—for their hard labor and for their firm and indomitable will displayed in overcoming one difficulty after another, and for their great success achieved in this way. As a leader in the circles of TCM, I am duty-bound to do my best to support them.

I believe this encyclopedia will be certain to find its position both in the history of Chinese medicine and in the history of world science and technology.

Mr. Zhang Qiwen
Member of the Standing Committee of All-China
Association of TCM, Deputy Head of the Health
Department of Shandong Province

Preface

English-Chinese Encyclopedia of Practical Traditional Chinese Medicine is an extensive series of twenty-one volumes. Based on the fundamental theories of Traditional Chinese Medicine(TCM) and with emphasis on the clinical practice of TCM, it is a semi-advanced English-Chinese academic work that is quite comprehensive, systematic, concise, practical, and easy to read. It caters mainly to the following readers: senior students of colleges of TCM, young and middle-aged teachers of colleges of TCM, young and middle-aged physicians of hospitals of TCM, personnel of scientific research institutions of TCM, teachers giving correspondence courses in TCM to foreigners, TCM personnel going abroad in the capacity of lecturers or physicians, those trained in Western medicine but wishing to study TCM, and foreigners coming to China to learn TCM or to take refresher courses in TCM.

Because Traditional Chinese Medicine and Pharmacology (TCMP) is unique to our Chinese nation, putting TCMP into English has been the crux of the compilation and translation of this encyclopedia. Since virtually no one can be proficient in the theories of Traditional Chinese Medicine and Pharmacology, the clinical practice of every branch of TCM, and English, collective translation measures have been taken to ensure that the English versions accurately express the inherent meanings of TCM. That is, teachers of English familiar with TCM, professional medical translators, teachers or physicians of TCM, and even teachers of paleography with a strong command of English were all invited together to co-translate the Chinese manuscripts and to then co-deliberate and discuss the English versions.

Finally, English-speaking foreigners studying TCM or teaching English in China were asked to polish the English versions. In this way, the skills of the above translators and foreigners were merged to ensure the quality of the English versions. However, even using this method, the uncertainty that the English versions will be wholly accepted still remains. As for the Chinese manuscripts, they do reflect the essence— and give a general picture—of traditional Chinese medicine and pharmacology. It is not asserted, though, that they are perfect. I wholeheartedly look forward to any criticisms or opinions from readers in order to make improvements to future editions. More than 200 people have taken part in the activities of compiling, translating, and revising this encyclopedia. They come from twenty-eight institutions in all parts of China. Among these institutions, there are fifteen colleges of TCM (Shandong, Beijing, Shanghai, Tianjin, Nanjing, Zhejiang, Anhui, Henan, Hubei, Guangxi, Guiyang, Gansu, Chengdu, Shanxi, and

Changchun) and scientific research centers of TCM such as China Academy of TCM and Shandong Scientific Research Institute of TCM.

The Education Commission of Shandong province has included the compilation and translation of this encyclopedia in its scientific research projects and allocated funds accordingly. The Health Department of Shandong Province has also given financial aid together with a number of pharmaceutical factories of TCM. The subsidization from Jinan Pharmaceutical Factory of TCM provided the impetus for the work of compilation and translation to get underway. The success of compiling and translating this encyclopedia is not only the fruit of the collective labor of all the compilers, translators, and revisers but also the result of the support of the responsible leaders of the relevant leading institutions. As the encyclopedia is going to be published, I express my heartfelt thanks to all the compilers, translators, and revisers for their sincere cooperation and to the specialists, professors, and leaders at all levels, as well as the pharmaceutical factories of TCM, for their warm support.

It is my most profound wish that the publication of this encyclopedia will take its role in cultivating talented persons of TCM having a very good command of TCM English and in extending, rapidly, comprehensive knowledge of TCM to all corners of the globe.

Xu Xiangcai
Shandong College of TCM

Introduction

Traditional Chinese Medicine (TCM) is one of China's great cultural heritages. Since the founding of the People's Republic of China in 1949 and guided by the farsighted TCM policy of the Chinese Communist Party and the Chinese government, the treasure house of the theories of TCM has been continuously explored, and the plentiful literature researched and compiled. As a result, great success has been achieved. Today, there has appeared a worldwide upsurge in the studying researching of TCM.

To promote even more vigorous development of this trend so that TCM may better serve all mankind, efforts are required to further it throughout the world. To bring this about, the language barriers must be overcome as soon as possible in order that TCM can be accurately expressed in foreign languages. Thus the compilation and translation of a series of English-Chinese books of basic knowledge of TCM has become of great urgency to serve the needs of medical and educational circles both inside and outside China.

In recent years, at the request of the health departments, satisfactory achievements have been made in researching the expression of TCM in English. Based on the investigation into the history and current state of the research work mentioned above, English-Chinese Encyclopedia of Practical Traditional Chinese Medicine has been published to meet the needs of extending the knowledge of TCM around the world. The encyclopedia consists of twenty-one volumes, each dealing with a particular branch of TCM. In the process of compilation, the distinguishing features of TCM have been given close attention, and great efforts have been made to ensure that the content is scientific, practical, comprehensive, and concise.

The chief writers of the Chinese manuscripts include professors or associate professors with at least twenty years of practical clinical and/or teaching experience in TCM. The Chinese manuscript of each volume has been checked and approved by a specialist of the relevant branch of TCM. The team of the translators and revisers of the English versions consists of TCM specialists with a good command of English professional medical translators and teachers of English from TCM colleges or universities.

At a symposium to standardize the English versions, scholars from twenty-two colleges and universities, research institutes of TCM, and other health institutes probed the question of how to express TCM in English more comprehensively, systematically, and accurately. They discussed and deliberated in detail the English versions of some volumes in order to upgrade the English versions of the whole series. The English version of each volume was re-examined and then given a final check.

Obviously this encyclopedia will provide extensive reading material of TCM English for senior students in colleges of TCM in China and will also greatly benefit foreigners studying TCM. The responsible leaders of the State Education Commission of the People's Republic of China, the State Administrative Bureau of TCM and Pharmacy, and the Education Commission and Health Department of Shandong Province have supported the assiduous efforts of compiling and translating this encyclopedia. Under the direction of the Higher Education Department of the State Education Commission, the leading board of compilation and translation of this encyclopedia was set up. The leaders of many colleges of TCM and pharmaceutical factories of TCM have also given assistance. We hope that this encyclopedia will positively enhance the teaching of TCM English at the colleges of TCM in China, on cultivating skills in medical circles to exchange ideas of TCM with patients in English, and on giving an impetus to the study of TCM outside China.

CHAPTER 1

An Introduction to Qigong for Treating Common Ailments

1.1 Concepts and Characteristics

Qigong is a psychosomatic regime, which through mind, breathing and posture regulation aids in the prevention and treatment of diseases as and preserves and lengthens life.

Qigong cultivates intrinsic energy (genuine Qi) which is found naturally within all people. Traditional Chinese medicine (TCM) holds that genuine Qi is a dynamic force, which powers all the vital functions in the human body.

There are many different forms of Qigong practice, each with its own distinct style and goals. *Daoyin*, also called *Daoyin* Massage, is a comprehensive exercise that combines specific body posture, breath regulation, and mind concentration with self-massage to develop both the physical and energetic aspects of the body. Inner Health Cultivation Exercise *(Neiyang Gong)*, Health Promotion Exercise *(Qiangzhuang Gong)*, Qi Nourishing Exercise *(Yangqi Gong)*, and Qi Circulation Exercise *(Zhoutian Gong)* are more specific Qigong methods which emphasize the training of genuine Qi. Regional *Daoyin* Exercise *(Buwei Daoyin Gong)*, and Five Viscera Regulation Exercise *(Li Wuzang Gong)* represent examples of Qigong exercises that focus their activity on specific areas of the body or on overcoming a specific disease.

Qigong exercises are chosen to meet the specific needs and conditions of its practitioner. When a Qigong method is selected, two aspects must be taken into consideration: the general improvement of the body functions as a whole and the treatment of an illness in particular. For example, Static Qigong, an exercise aimed at training and accumulating Qi, builds up the constitution and obtains longevity. It is excellent for improving a generally healthy body. On the other hand, for someone who is already sick, it is desirable to pick a Qigong exercise optimal to aid in the treatment of the specific disease. For example, people having palpitations and shortness of breath due to insufficiency of the heart Qi may practice Heart Regulation Exercise *(Lixin Gong)* to achieve rapid therapeutic effects. In TCM, the selection and practice of Qigong according to the constitution of individuals and the nature of their illnesses is called Differential Diagnosis and Treatment.

Qigong emphasizes the cultivation of health through the removal of all blockages in the mind and body. As observed by the ancient Chinese, running water never turns stale and a door hinge never gets worm-eaten. *Daoying An Qiao*, an exercise found in *The Yellow Emperor's Canon of Internal Medicine (Huang Di Nei Jing)*, consists mainly of self-massage and self-controlled movements of the extremities to build up the constitution, to guide Qi and blood circulation and to control diseases. Like all Qigong, this exercise is to a great extent superior to the passive methods of massage, acupuncture, drug medication and other therapies in its ability to mobilize the vital energy to prevent and cure diseases. Other advantages of Qigong are its simplicity and feasibility. It can be learned, with rapid and satisfactory results by reading books with illustrations.

1.2 The Development of Qigong

Qigong, as an art of healing and health preservation, is thought to have originated as early as four thousand years ago in the *Tang Yao* times as a form of dancing. *Lu's Spring and Autumn Annals* or *Lu's History (Lu Shi Chun Qiu)* records, In the beginning of the Tao Tang Tribes, the sun was often shut off by heavy clouds and it rained all the time; turbulent waters overflowed the rivers' banks. People lived a gloomy and dull life and suffered from rigidity of their joints. As a remedy dancing was recommended. From the experience of their long-term struggle with nature, the ancients gradually realized that body movements, exclamations and various ways of breathing could help readjust certain bodily functions. For example, imitating animal movements such as climbing, looking about, and leaping was found to promote a vital flow of Qi. Pronouncing "Hi" was found to either decrease or increase strength, "Ha" could disperse heat, and "Xu" could alleviate pain. In this way, Qigong was brought into being.

During the Spring and Autumn and the Warring States Periods (770-221 B.C.), various schools of thought arose such schools rationalized and raised to the level of theory their knowledge of nature, society and life based on the experiences of their predecessors. Through this process, Qigong found its way to systematization and became an independent theoretical construct popular with philosophers and scholars. The theories of Qigong continued to develop and coalesce into powerful new concepts such as the three treasures of the human body (life essence, Qi, and mental faculties). Qigong methods also started to develop during this time. "Exhale and inhale to expel the stale and take in the fresh", "a bear twists its neck", or "a bird stretches its wings," are a few examples of such methods.

The Qin (221–207 B.C.) and Han (206 B. C.-A.D. 220) dynasties saw a rapid development of medical skills, which in turn enhanced Qigong theory and practice. *The Yellow Emperor's Canon of Internal Medicine*, the earliest medical classic extant in China, described *Daoyin*, Guidance of Qi, and *An Qiao* as important curative measures that could also preserve life. It also offered the following advice, which besides offering a general life philosophy, describes the state of mind necessary for successful Qigong practice: "Be indifferent to fame or gain, be alone in repose, and take the various parts of the body as an organic whole." There is an account of *Daoyin* found in *Plain Questions On Acupuncture (Su Wen Yi Pian Ci Fa Lun)* that says, "Patients with lingering kidney disease may face south from 3 to 5 A.M., concentrate the mind, hold back the breath, crane the neck and swallow Qi as if swallowing a hard object seven times. After that, there would be a great amount of fluid welling up from under the tongue." In 1973, a silk book, *Fasting and Taking Qi (Que Gu Shi Qi Pian)* and a silk painting *Daoyin Chart (Dao Yin Tu)* of the Western Han dynasty (206 B.C.-A.D. 24) were unearthed from the Han Dynasty Tomb Mawangdui No. 3 in Changsha, Hunan Province. The book records the *Daoyin* method for guiding Qi and the chart covers 44 colored paintings presenting human figures imitating the movements of a wolf, monkey, ape, bear, crane, hawk, and vulture. Thus, they reveal that the Chinese began to teach Qigong pictorially as early as the beginning of the Western Han dynasty. The two outstanding medical scholars Zhang Zhongjing and Hua Tuo, in the closing years of the Eastern Han dynasty (A.D. 25–220), both aided in the development of Qigong. In his great work, *Synopsis of the Prescriptions of the Golden Chamber (Jin Kui Yao Luo)*, Zhang Zhongiing stated that "As soon as heaviness and sluggishness of the extremities is felt, start *Daoyin*, breathing exercises, acupuncture, moxibustion, and massage with application of ointment to prevent obstruction of the nine orifices." The famous exercise Frolics of Five Animals (*Wu Qin Xi*) was devised during this time by Hua Tuo and became widely practiced and it is still popular today.

During the Wei dynasty (A.D. 220–265), the Jin dynasty (A.D. 265–420), and the Northern and Southern dynasties (A.D. 420–589), Qigong developed as a way of preserving health and as a method for treating disease through the emission of Qi. Zhang Zhan of the Jin dynasty listed in his work *Yang Sheng Essentials of Health Preservation (Yao Ji)* ten essential practices, of which thrifty of mentality, preservation of Qi, conservation of constitution, and *Daoyin* were all related to Qigong. Tao Hongjing of the Northern and Southern dynasties recorded in his book, *Health Preservation and Longevity (Yang Sheng Yan Ming Lu)*, many ancient Qigong methods and theories. In *The History of the Jin Dynasty (Jin Shu)*, there is an account of doctor Xing Ling who became famous for using outgoing Qi to cure a patient who had suffered more than ten years from flaccidity arthralgia syndrome. As a result of this success, many more people became interested in medical Qigong.

Qigong was widely put into clinical application in the Sui (A.D. 581–618) the Tang (A.D. 618–907) dynasties. The books *General Treatise on the Causes and Symptoms of Diseases (Zhu Bing Yuan Hou Lun)*, *Prescriptions Worth a Thousand Gold for Emergencies (Bei Ji Qian Jin YaoFang)* and *The Medical Secrets of Official (Wai Tai Mi Yao)* contain a wealth of Qigong therapies for treating specific pathologies. *The General Treatise on the Cause and Symptoms of Diseases*, records more than 260 Qigong therapies, The *Brahman Method* of Indian Massage and *Laozi* Massage along with other Qigong *Daoyin* massage methods of health preservation in the text, *Prescriptions Worth a Thousand Gold for Emergencies*. *Master Huan Zhen's Knacks in Taking Qi (Huan Zhen Xian Sheng Fu Nei Zhi Qi Jue)* of the Tang dynasty describes the *Pithy Formulae of Qi Distribution*, which introduces the essential principles and techniques for emitting outgoing Qi.

During the period of the Song (A.D. 960–1279), Jin (A.D. 1115–1234), and Yuan (A.D. 1271–1368) dynasties, an upsurge of Daoist exercises for cultivating spiritual energy Qigong began to merge with these exercises giving rise to more sophisticated forms of therapeutic Qigong. Within the book *The Complete Record of Holy Benevolence (Sheng Ji Zong Lu)* is a wealth of Qigong information. Many Qigong descriptions can also be found in the works of the four eminent physicians of the Jin and Yuan dynasties. Li Dongyuan wrote in his book, *Secret Record of the Chamber of Orchids (Lan Shi Mi Cang)*, "Falling ill, the patient should sit still at ease to replenish Qi." Liu Wansu mentioned, in his *Etiology Based on Plain Questions (Su Wen Xuan Ji Bing Yuan Shi)*, the application of the Six Character Formulae in the treatment of diseases.

Zhu Zhenheng stated in his book, *Danxi's Experiential Therapy (Dan Xi Xin Fa)*, that "Patients with syncope, flaccidity, or cold or heat syndrome due to stagnation of Qi should be treated with *Daoyin* exercises."

During the period of the Ming (A.D. 1368–1644) and Qing (A.D.1644–1911) dynasties, doctors characterized the development of Qigong by deeper mastery and wider application. This enriched the medical books with Qigong literature and data. Abundant Qigong information was included in several influential books: *A Retrospective Collection of Medical Classics (Yi Jing Su Hui Ji)* by Wang Lu, *Wanmizhai's Ten Categories of Medical Works (Wan Mi Zhai Yi Shu Shi Zhong)* by Wan Quan, and *The General Medicine of the Past and Present (Gu Jin Yi Tong Da Quan)* compiled by Xu Chunpu. The great physician Li Shizhen stated definitively in his book, *A Study on the Eight Extra Channels (Qi Jing Ba Mai Kao)*, that "The internal conditions and the channels can only be perceived by those who can see things by inward vision." This famous thesis indicated the relationship between Qigong and the channels and collaterals.

Qigong has gained higher priority and more rapid development since the founding of the People's Republic of China. In 1955, a Qigong hospital was established in Tangshan. During this time two important books introduced exercises such as internal cultivation, keep-fit, and many others, thus, giving an impetus to the development of Qigong research throughout the whole country. These books are *The Practice of Qigong Therapy (Liao Fa Shi Jian)* written by Liu Guizhen *and Qigong and Keep-fit Qigong (Qi Gong Ji Bao Jian Qi Gong)* written by Hu Yaozhen. Since 1978, medical workers and Qigong masters all over China have made vigorous efforts to popularize Qigong for health preservation and disease prevention. Some scientists and technicians have not only studied Qigong in terms of physiology, biochemistry and modern medicine, but they have also conducted multi-disciplinary research efforts to analyze the physical effect of outgoing Qi. A study on the nature and essence of Qigong has thus been initiated, and Qigong, as a new branch of science, has entered a period of vigorous development. Qigong research societies, hospitals and departments have been established to research, teach and use Qigong. Qigong practice and study have become commonplace throughout China. Over the last 12 years, many Qigong journals and magazines have been published. Journals include: *The Journal of Qigong (Qi Gong Za Zhi)*, *Qigong and Science (Qi Gong Yu Ke Xue)*, *China Qigong (Zhong Hua Qi Gong)*, *Chinese Qigong (Zhong Guo Qi Gong)*, and *Orient Qigong (Dong Fang Qi Gong)*. Qigong books include: *Outstanding Examples of Qigong Therapy (Qi Gong Liao Fa Ji Jin)*, *New Qigong Therapy (Xin Qi Gong Liao Fo)*, *The Science of Chinese Qigong (Zhong Guo Qi Gong Xue)*, and *Principles of Qigong Regime (Qi Gong Yang Sheng Xue Gai Yao)*.

1.3 Basic Principles of Qigong

1.3.1 BEING BOTH DYNAMIC AND STATIC

"Dynamic" and "static" are two general terms used in Qigong to differentiate Qigong practices. Methods that require limb and body movements are referred to as dynamic Qigong. Qigong methods that require little or no physical movement are referred to as static Qigong. Qigong exercises are selected to suit the health status of the individual practitioner. The practice of static Qigong is aimed at accumulating Qi in the *Diantian*, and with further practice, to circulate Qi throughout all of the meridians in the body. *Daoyin* and dynamic Qigong aims to promote the free flow of Qi in the meridians, muscles and skeleton as well as to alleviate specific areas of physical energetic congestion that manifest as disease. Regardless of which of the two Qigong forms is practiced, the principle "cherish stillness in motion and motion in stillness" should be adhered to. When *Daoyin* or dynamic Qigong is practiced, keep a serene, concentrated mind throughout the movements. When static Qigong is practiced, keep the body relaxed throughout the mental stimulation of the meridians and collaterals.

1.3.2 BEING RELAXED AND NATURAL

When practicing Qigong, relaxation must be both physical and mental. However, relaxation does not mean slackness or inattentiveness. Instead, it refers to a balance between tension and suppleness dominated by the conscious mind. A major goal of Qigong is to re-establish a natural harmony between being and moving which often gets lost through daily activity. In this state of harmony there will be no tension, but the energy within the body will be activated and the mind will be fully engaged.

1.3.3 COORDINATING THE WILL AND QI

In Qigong exercise, the will and Qi should move together. The practitioner should not put undue emphasis on breathing mechanics (i.e., gentle, fine, even and long) other than what is acquired naturally through correct practice. Abdominal respiration, which requires bulging of the belly and protruding the chest, should be avoided at the beginning. Attention to natural motion must be given and the flow of

Qi should not be forced in a particular direction. Yue Yanggui of the Qing dynasty (A.D. 1644–1911) wrote in his book *Questions and Answers of Meihua (Meihua Wen Da Pian)*, that "the tranquility of the mind regulates the breathing naturally and, in turn, regulated breathing brings on concentration of the mind naturally." This is what is meant by, "the mind and breathing are interdependent and regular respiration produces a serene mind." It is also not advisable to put undue emphasis the flow of Qi. The cold, hot, tingling, distending, itching, light, heavy, floating, deep, or warm sensations that one can experience during Qigong exercise will often go along a specific route. It is improper to pursue a specific sensation intentionally, to exaggerate it, or to force oneself to gain it. When practicing *Daoyin* Qigong self-massage, it is stipulated that the will should follow the hand manipulations so as to realize the feeling of Qi under the hands. If the feeling is not quite tangible, one should not pursue it recklessly. It is enough just to concentrate the attention on the site under the hands.

1.3.4 COMBINING ACTIVE EXERCISE WITH INNER HEALTH CULTIVATION

Active exercise refers to a series of procedures used to expel distracting thoughts, regulate respiration, attain proper posture, and relax both mind and body. Active exercise requires control of consciousness by means of breathing and will. It may even involve hand manipulations.

Inner health cultivation refers to the quiet state one falls into after active exercise. In this state, one feels relaxed and comfortable; the will and breathing is quiet.

Qigong active exercise and inner health cultivation are done alternately and promote each other. For instance, one may perform static inner health cultivation immediately after practicing *Daoyin*, or vice versa, to achieve the effectiveness of active exercise in static cultivation or static cultivation in active exercise. By using both together, one can rapidly achieve a high level of Qigong.

1.3.5 PROCEEDING STEP BY STEP

Qigong should be practiced in an orderly way. When Qigong or *Daoyin* is practiced, priority should be given to the selection of practice methods. Be aware of the old saying, "Haste makes waste." Through arduous training, the practitioner will be able to direct Qi to follow changes in body posture, hand manipulations, respiration and will. It is essential to learn basic theories before beginning Qigong practice. Common errors are: eagerness to achieve quick results, trying to cure an illness overnight, and too much practice leading to fatigue, pain, soreness or exacerbation of an illness. Slackness, carelessness, and sloppiness in practice are also common impediments to successful Qigong practice. Those who let things drift, chop and change, go fishing for three days and dry the nets for two will be unable to develop true Qigong ability. Therefore, to succeed in Qigong exercise, one needs to adhere to the requirements and practice earnestly. Efforts should be made to overcome all objective difficulties. If one is conversant with Qigong knowledge and practices the exercises with perseverance, results are guaranteed.

CHAPTER 2

The Three Regulations

2.1 Regulation of the Body (Adjustment of Posture)

Regulation of the body is also called posturization or adjustment of posture. It is especially important for the beginners of *Daoyin* or static Qigong to have a good command of this skill. In Qigong exercise, four basic postures may be assumed; they are: sitting, lying, standing and walking. Static Qigong usually requires a sitting, lying or standing posture, while *Daoyin* can be practiced using all four.

2.1.1 SITTING POSTURES

There are two sitting postures addressed in this text: upright sitting and sitting cross-legged.

Upright Sitting. Sit upright on a large, even, square stool. Place the feet parallel to each other at a distance as wide as the shoulders. Bend the knees to form an angle of 90 degrees. Keep the trunk erect so that it forms a 90 degree angle with the thighs. Rest the palms gently on the thighs. Bend the arms at the elbows naturally and look straight ahead. Tuck in the chin a little and let down the shoulders, drawing in the chest slightly inward to keep the back straight. Close the eyes and mouth. Touch the tip of the tongue to the palate (Fig. 1).

Sitting Cross-legged. Sit on something soft with your legs crossed beneath you so that the foot of one leg rests beneath the other leg. Place a cushion under the hips to raise them a little causing the body to lean slightly forward. Grasp the hands in front of the abdomen with the left above the right. With the thumb of the right hand, press *Ziwen* (located at the union of the palm and the ring finger) of the left hand, and join the thumb and the middle finger of the left hand together (Fig. 2).

2.1.2 LYING DOWN POSTURES

There are two lying down postures addressed within this text, lateral recumbent posture and supine posture.

Lateral Recumbent Posture. Lie down (usually on the left side but either side will do) and bend the trunk slightly. Rest the head on a pillow and tilt it slightly towards the chest. Keep the eyes and mouth slightly closed and the tongue against the palate. Stretch the leg of the

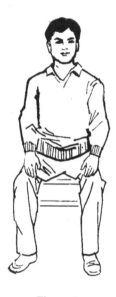

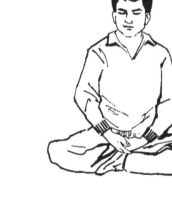

Figure 1   Figure 2

lower side naturally, bend the top leg and rest it naturally on the lower one. Place the hand of the lower side comfortably on the pillow with the palm facing upwards, and place the hand of the upper side naturally on the hip (Fig. 3).

Supine Posture. Lie on your back with the face upward and the neck straight. Place the two hands at the sides of the body or on the abdomen, overlapping one another. Keep the eyes and mouth slightly closed and the tongue against the palate (Fig. 4).

2.1.3 STANDING POSTURE

Set the feet shoulder-width apart. Keep the head straight and the trunk erect with the chest bent slightly inward. Keep the knees at ease and the arms raised and bent a little. Keep the fingers apart naturally, and hold the two hands close to the chest or the lower abdomen as if holding a ball (Fig. 5). The standing posture can be varied in several ways.

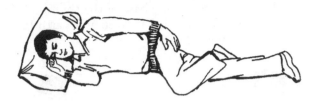

Figure 3

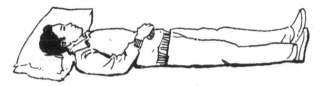

Figure 4

- The palms may be in front of the body facing downward (Fig.6)
- The palms may be overlapped in front of the lower abdomen (Fig.7)
- The right arm may bend in front of the chest with the palm upward and level with the acupuncture point Tanzhong (Ren 17), while the left hand is held erect with the fingers pointing

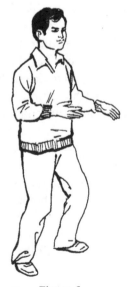

Figure 5

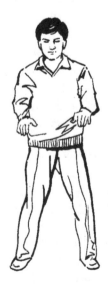

Figure 6

11

upward and the palm facing the base of the thumb of the right hand. This last position is called Heaven and Earth Palms (*Qiankun Zhang* gesture) (Fig.8)

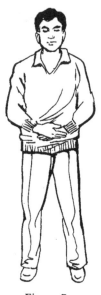

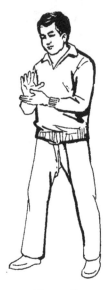

Figure 7   Figure 8

2.1.4 POSTURE ESSENTIALS

Concerning the requirements for posture in Qigong, *The Eight Annotations on Health Preservation (Zun Sheng Ba Jian)* cites a quotation from *The Book on Mentality (Xin Shu)*, saying "Sit on a thick-padded cushion, loosen the clothing, keep the back straight up, get the lips close to the teeth and prop the tongue against the palate, keep the eyes slightly open and stare at the apex of the nose." Although there are a variety of postures in Qigong exercise, the essential requirements are the same for all of them:

1. Loosen the clothes. This step is essential to ensure a smooth flow of Qi through channels and collaterals.

2. Image that an object is being supported on the head (called Suspending the Crown of the Head). This protocol helps keep the head upright, the chin slightly tucked, and neck lifted a little so it is straight and relaxed.

3. Relax the shoulders and drop the elbows. This should be done with ease, avoiding stiffness of the elbows.

4. Draw in the chest and straighten the back. The practitioner should not over-relax the back or lean it against anything.

Instead, the chest should be drawn in slightly which naturally keeps the back in proper position.

5. Keep the waist and the abdomen relaxed. The waist and abdomen are vital for proper training and guiding of Qi. The abdomen is usually described as the furnace for refining vital energy. The waist is the residence of the kidneys (the repository of original Qi) and the gate of life (an energetic construct between the kidneys) and is therefore an important source of Qi and blood circulation.

6. Contract the buttocks and relax the knees slightly. Contracting the hips helps to straighten the spinal column; relaxing the knees permits free flow of Qi through the Three Yang and Three Yin Channels of the Foot.

7. Keep the toes clutching the ground. When the standing posture is taken, stretch the feet and let the five toes of each foot clutch the ground to keep the body as firm as Mount Tai (as stable as possible).

8. Drop the eyelids (called Curtain-falling and Inward Vision). This name refers to a method of dropping the eyelids to create inward vision on the spot where Qi is trained or circulated.

   The book Yin Fu Jing claims that the functional activities of the body are influenced by the eyes; Miraculous Pivot the 2nd part of Canon of Medicine (Ling Shu Jing) holds that the eyes are the messengers of the mind, and the mind is the home of vitality. Eyes are of great importance in Qigong exercise. Curtain-falling and Inward Vision help keep the mind undisturbed, guarding against hallucination and distracting light. The eyes should neither be tightly closed nor left wide open. In the former, drowsiness may occur because of darkness and, in the latter, vitality may be disturbed because of too much light.

9. Close the mouth and stop the ears. Laozi (Laotzi) once said, "Close the mouth to shut the gate." Closing the mouth here refers to closing the mouth slightly without clenching the teeth or tightening the lips. Stopping the ears means to focus one's hearing to oneself so as to be free from outside interference (also called Inward-hearing).

10. Sticking the tongue against the palate (called Propping the Palate with the Tongue Tip or Tongue Propping). It is a way of placing the tongue naturally against the palate so communication is established between the Ren and Du Channels (two major channels which transverse the front (Yen) and back (Yu) of the body. In the course of practice, the strength of the

tongue sticking against the palate will increase automatically, and the tongue body will be gradually pulled backward. This is a phenomenon occurring in the course of Qigong practice and should not be pursued intentionally.

When *Daoyin* is practiced, adjustment of the posture, and hand manipulation methods such as pushing, rubbing, and kneading should be carried out with ease. Rigidity in movement should be avoided.

2.2 Regulation of Breathing

Regulation of breathing, also called inhaling and exhaling, breathing method, venting or taking in, is an important link in Qigong exercise. The ancients attached great importance to breathing exercises and described a great number of methods including: inhaling *(Fu-Qi)*, eating *(Shi-Qi)*, entering *(Jin-Qi)*, swallowing *(Yan-Qi)*, circulating *(Xing-Qi)*, taking in *(Cai-Qi)*, upper breathing *(Shang-Xi)*, lower breathing *(Xia-Xi)*, full breathing *(Mun-Xi)*, blurted breathing *(Chong-Xi)*, lasted breathing *(Chi-Xi)*, long breathing *(Chang-Xi)*, and deep breathing *(Shen-Xi)*. The breathing methods described in the following sections are the ones most commonly used in Qigong practice.

2.2.1 NATURAL RESPIRATION

Natural respiration is the ordinary breathing pattern that occurs under normal physical conditions. Because of the difference in physiology between male and female and the difference in the breathing habits of individuals, natural respiration can be further divided into natural thoracic respiration, natural abdominal respiration, and a combination of the two. Breathing techniques should be relaxed and performed naturally. Natural respiration is the most commonly used Qigong breathing method, especially for beginners.

2.2.2 ABDOMINAL RESPIRATION

Abdominal respiration also known as abdominal breathing is developed gradually under the guidance of the will until it occurs naturally. To train abdominal respiration, one uses the consciousness to relax the abdominal muscles so that the abdomen expands naturally during inspiration and contracts during exhalation. The contraction and relaxation of the abdominal muscles are intensified gradually and naturally through practice. Forced exertion must be avoided.

2.2.3 REVERSE ABDOMINAL RESPIRATION

Reverse abdominal respiration is the main breathing method used in advanced Qigong exercises and during the emission of outgoing Qi. In this method, one uses the will to contract the abdominal muscles during inspiration and to relax them so that the abdomen expands during expiration. Although this method is initially awkward, it will become natural through proper training. When reverse abdominal respiration becomes more or less natural, it can be done in cooperation with contraction of the anus, which increases the physical and energetic force of the movement.

2.2.4 OTHER BREATHING METHODS

Apart from the methods mentioned above, there is also long inhaling and short exhaling, long exhaling and short inhaling, nasal expiration and nasal inspiration, nasal inspiration and oral expiration, and respiratory pause after expiration or inspiration. The selection of the breathing method is based on the goal of a particular Qigong exercise and the level of the practitioner. Each exercise in this book includes a clear description of its associated breathing strategy.

2.2.5 ESSENTIALS OF RESPIRATION TRAINING

It is preferable to focus on developing correct posture when one begins practicing dynamic Qigong, *Daoyin*, or static Qigong. Training of respiration should begin after one is skilled and natural in posturing. Adverse effects, such as respiratory distress, emotional upset, chest stuffiness, and headache, may result when breathing techniques are used in conjunction with an improper Qigong posture. The final goal of respiration training is to achieve deep, long, even and fine respiration as the result of long-term practice. Forced movements with lengthened or oppressed breath should be avoided.

When practicing *Daoyin* exercises, the movement of the hands is often done in cooperation with the respiration. For example, pushing along the inner arm (Three *Yin* Channels of Hands) towards the fingertips is accompanied by expiration and pushing along the outer arm (Three *Yang* Channels of Hand) towards the shoulders and head is accompanied by inspiration. The direction of movement is often based on the way the Qi flows through the body.

Before starting respiration training, it is desirable to perform the following cleansing exercise. Open the mouth and imagine that turbid Qi and matter are being dredged from the obstructed parts of all the vessels and expelled from the body through expiration. Close the mouth and imagine that fresh air is filling the entire body during inhalation. Repeat the above exercise three times and then breathe naturally. Gradually adjust to the respiration requirements of the chosen Qigong exercise that will be practiced next.

2.3 Regulation of Mental Activities

Regulation of mental activities is also known as will control or thinking method. The training of the will is the most important link in Qigong exercise. *The Three Gists of Regime (Sheng San Yao)* says, "Preservation of the essence of life rests with cultivation of vital energy, which in turn rests with mental faculties. Mental faculty to vital energy is as mother is to child. Thus, concentration of the mind would have vital energy consolidated while distraction of the mind would have it dispersed. One who only tries to save essence of life but neglects mental faculty knows the how but does not know the why." This passage stresses the relationship between essence of life, vital energy, and mental faculty and points out the primary function of mental activities in Qigong practice.

2.3.1 BASIC STRATEGIES FOR REGULATING THE MIND

There are various strategies used to regulate the mind during Qigong practice. The type of mind regulation used is dependent on the particular Qigong exercise being practiced.

Localized mind concentration is concentration of the mind on a certain part or point of the body, such as the upper, middle, or lower *Dantian*, the acupuncture points *Yongquan* (K 1) and *Laogong* (P 8), the fingertips or palms, or on a spot fixed outside the body. Directive Mind Concentration occurs when the flow of Qi is sensed when the mind goes with the movement of the hands or with internal movements of the channels. Rhythmical Mind Concentration focuses the mind on repetition, like the vibration produced by driving a pile. It occurs rhythmically, or moves slowly with normal respiratory cycles. During Qigong practice, one may imagine attaining superhuman strength. For example, one may imagine that he or she is strong enough to push a hill, hold up the sky, or pull nine oxen back by the tails. This kind of mind concentration is called Power-Strengthening Mind Concentration. Coordination of thought, movement, and language is known as Suggestive Mind Concentration. It includes saying words silently and meditating on the results you wish to achieve by Qigong exercise. Representative Mind Concentration requires the practitioner to imagine a particular movement in order to stimulate the flow of Qi. For instance, one may imagine stroking or pressing a ball; expelling unhealthy Qi; or feeling as hot as fire, as cold as ice, as sharp as a sword, or as soft as cotton.

2.3.2 ESSENTIALS OF TRAINING MENTAL ACTIVITIES

Mental activities should be coordinated naturally with respiration and posture. Mental activities should be carried out naturally and progressively in a composed state of mind. The training of mental activity cannot go without confidence. No matter what kind of mental activity you are exercising, you should be confident that the goal will be attained, although you should not expect quick results. If something unexpected happens during the process, do not be overjoyed or frightened.

2.4 Points for Attention in Qigong Exercise

If Qigong exercises are to be practiced successfully, it is essential for beginners to clearly understand the movements, breathing methods, mental activities, and main theories of the exercises. Manipulation methods should be selected properly and the acupuncture points should be spotted correctly. Practicing Qigong with maximum effort should only occur after one is well acquainted with all of the basics. One must have clear goals, be confident and determined, and persevere. The Qigong exercises must be practiced step by step. One's work, study, and life activities should be arranged properly so as to avoid distracting thoughts and anxiety during practice. It is best to practice Qigong in a quiet place where fresh air is readily available. Avoid practicing the exercises in a draft, near a fan or air conditioner. In order to avoid any possible disturbance to the functional activities of Qi and the circulation of blood, one should first set his mind at rest, relieve oneself, loosen the belt and remove the watch and spectacles. If practicing *Daoyin*, the areas of the body that need to be manipulated should be exposed. It is advisable to practice according to the established time requirements associated with each exercise. The overall time for Qigong exercise is flexible and should be set in accordance with the practitioner's constitution and the severity of one's illness. One should not force oneself to prolong the exercise time or to increase the frequency. An optimum frequency and duration will always leave one with energy and interest and not tiredness. Qigong practice should be avoided after eating too much or when hungry. Practicing one hour after eating is desirable. For the purpose of curing diseases comprehensive measures should be taken, and Qigong may be performed in combination with medication or other therapies. If practicing during menstruation, the time for exercise should not be too long and excessive and concentration on the lower part of the body should be avoided. During Qigong practice, some sensations such as heat, distention, aching, tingling or numbness, itching, coolness, muscle twitch, or a sensation of bugs crawling on the body may occur. These are the normal manifestations of the functional activities of Qi. One should neither be nervous or frightened, nor attempt to feel them. Just let things take their own course. When Qigong is practiced, sexual intercourse, smoking, drinking, and intake of tea and hot or acid food should be moderate. Try to give up smoking gradually.

If you are suddenly panic-stricken during exercise by a loud sound, unexpected interruption, or peculiar phenomena, do not be nervous. Try to find out the cause of the panic, set the mind at ease, and then continue the exercises. Qigong exercise needs a steady start, steady performance, and steady ending. Carelessness may result in failure to conduct Qi back to its origin or cause disorder of the functional activities of the body. Treatment of patients by emitting Qi should only be performed by those who have sufficient training and experience.

CHAPTER 3

Various Qigong Exercises

3.1 Psychosomatic Relaxation Exercise *(Fangsong Gong)*

Functions: Relaxes internal and external aspects of the body, develops the skill necessary to practice advanced Qigong.

Psychosomatic relaxation is a basic exercise, which is easier to master than other forms of static Qigong. One must be relaxed, quiet, and natural no matter which Qigong exercise is being practiced. Certain types of psychosomatic relaxation serve to initiate practitioners into more serious Qigong exercises.

Methods

The standing, sitting, and lying postures are all appropriate for psychosomatic relaxation. No matter what posture is taken, the principle of being relaxed, quiet, and natural should always be remembered. The muscles, connective tissue, organs, and mind should be as relaxed as possible. The eyes can be either gently closed or slightly open.

1. **Three-line Relaxation.** The first line refers to the surface of the lateral sides of the head, neck, and shoulders. The second refers to the anterior surface of the face, neck, chest, abdomen, and lower limbs; the third includes the posterior surface of the head, neck, back, waist and the lower limbs. When doing the exercises, concentrate the mind on the first segment of the first line and silently say, "Relax." Sequentially repeat this technique for all the segments that make up the first line. When finished, proceed to the second and the third lines. Using natural respiration, repeat this cycle 3–5 times.

2. **Regional Relaxation.** Silently say, "Relax" while sequentially concentrating on the head, shoulders, upper limbs, back, waist, hips, and lower limbs. Repeat the procedure 3–5 times while breathing naturally.

3. **General Relaxation.** Slowly relax the whole body from the head down to the feet, as if taking a warm shower. Use natural respiration.

4. **Closing the Exercise.** End all activity associated with exercise and remain quiet for a while. To finish the exercise, gently rub the face and hands. One may also overlap the hands (the left under the right in male and vice versa in female) and rest them on the navel. Move the hands in a circular fashion clockwise for 36 turns. Gradually increase the size of the circle as you move outward from the navel to the flanks. Reverse this process and rotate the palms counterclockwise decreasing the size of the circle until returning to the navel. Rub the face and hands again to end the exercise.

Application

Psychosomatic relaxation is generally used for health preservation and as a Qigong exercise for beginners. It is also used for treating many chronic diseases such as hypertension, neurosis, bronchitis, bronchial asthma, menopausal syndrome, gastritis, gastric and duodenal ulcers, and chronic pelvic inflammation. Hypertension, headache, dizziness and other disorders are often treated with the Three-line Relaxation method in combination with the Head and Face Exercise described later in this manual. Diseases of the lung, stomach, and heart are usually allayed with the regional relaxation method by emphasizing the relaxation of the diseased parts.

Points for Attention

This exercise can be done 1–4 times a day. The type of psychosomatic relaxation used is determined by the conditions of the individual. Psychosomatic relaxation is usually done with natural respiration in coordination with mental activities (will). In general, the mind should be concentrated on a certain part of the body during inspiration, and the word "Relax" is said silently during expiration. Concentrating one's mind is a paradoxical activity in which it may seem that one is both thinking about and not thinking about a certain area of the body. It is natural for distraction to occur in the beginning. Keep lighthearted when doing this exercise. Stop the exercise temporarily whenever you become angry or overexcited. If you feel lethargic in a lying posture, try sitting or standing.

3.2 Inner Health Cultivation Exercise *(Ne jyang Gong)*

Functions: Combines silent recitation of words with breathing and also invigorates the functions of the digestive and respiratory systems.

Methods

This exercise utilizes either nasal respiration or oral-nasal breathing techniques.

1. **Nasal Respiration.** Assume a lying or sitting posture, and select either abdominal or reverse breathing. During nasal inspiration, put the tip of the tongue against the palate and direct Qi down to the *Dantian* (1.3 cm inferior to the navel), thinking the word "I". Hold the breath and silently say "keep", "I keep quiet", or "I keep quiet for the good of my health". During expiration, the tongue is released. At the beginning, use fewer words and slowly increase the number. For example, start with three, then five, and finally to nine words, the maximum. Inhale when you say the first part of the sentence and exhale when you say the second part. Hold the breath when you say the word in the middle.

2. **Oral-nasal Respiration.** Use abdominal respiration. Inhale though the nose and direct Qi down to the *Dantian*, exhale through the mouth. Hold the breath with the tongue stuck against the palate, while silently speaking the appropriate words as discussed above. Release the tongue when you finish the words and begin again for another round. End this exercise in the same way as Psychosomatic Relaxation Exercise.

Application

This exercise is indicated for prevention and treatment of chronic gastritis, gastric ulcer, duodenal ulcer, chronic hepatitis, neurosis, hypertension, irregular menstruation, dysmenorrhea, and other disorders.

Points for Attention

Practice of this exercise is recommended 1–4 times a day, 10–60 minutes each time. Use abdominal respiration at the initial stage of practice and change to reverse breathing when you are very familiar with the mechanics of this exercise. During the initial stages of the exercise, use no more that three words when holding the breath. As you become more comfortable with the practice, gradually increase the number of words you silently say. Do not force yourself to hold your breath or bulge your abdomen. A warm sensation will be felt in the lower abdomen after long-time practice.

3.3 Health Promotion Exercise (Qiangzhuang Gong)

Functions: Reinforces intrinsic Qi and promotes good health and the ability to prevent and cure disease.

Methods

Natural respiration or reverse breathing techniques can be used in the practice of this exercise.

1. **Natural Respiration.** Sit cross-legged or take a standing posture. Gradually regulate your breath so that it is quiet, even, fine, and slow. Concentrate the mind on the *Dantian.*

2. **Reverse Breathing.** Sit cross-legged or stand using reverse breathing while concentrating the mind on the *Dantian.* Pull in the abdomen and contract the anus during inspiration to pull Qi into the *Dantian.* Expand the abdomen during expiration to allow Qi to move throughout the entire body.

Application

Health Promotion Exercise improves health and treats hypertension, neurosis, coronary heart disease, and arthritis.

Points for Attention

This exercise can be practiced 1–4 times a day, 10–60 minutes each time. Fine, even, deep, and long respiration can only be achieved through long-term practice and should not be pursued forcefully or by suppressing breath. Stop exercising before you get tired.

3.4 Head and Face Exercise (Toumian Gong)

Functions: Promotes a clear complexion, prevents and treats diseases by adjusting the channels and acupuncture points on the head, and increases blood circulation.

Methods

1. **Preparation.** Take the upright sitting or standing posture. Relax the entire body, applying the tongue against the palate. Close the eyes slightly and get rid of distractions.

2. **Pushing the Forehead.** Put the index, middle, and ring fingers of each hand together. Push the forehead with the fingertips from the midpoint of the eyebrows upward to the front hairline 24–50 times (Fig.9) and from the

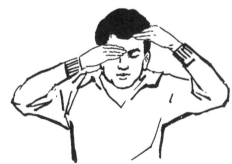

Figure 9

midpoint of the forehead outward toward the temples 24–50 times. The right hand should push the right side and the left hand should push the left. Respiration should be fine and long. Push with more force while exhaling and less while inhaling. Try to feel beneath your hands while pushing.

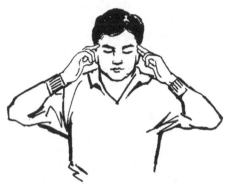

3. **Kneading Motion.** Put the middle fingers against the depression lateral to the external canthi (corner of the eye) on either side of the head (Acupuncture point *Taiyang* (Extra 2)). Press and knead in a counterclockwise motion 24–50 times (Fig. 10). Refer to method 2 (Pushing the Forehead) for

Figure 10

methods of mind concentration and respiration.

4. **Bathing the Face.** Rub the face with the two palms. Start from the midpoint of the forehead and move outward toward the hairline and ears, downward and then upward along the sides of the nose and back to the forehead. Rub clockwise with one palm and counterclockwise with another, and vice versa, 24–50 times using natural respiration. Try to get an electric feeling under the palms while rubbing.

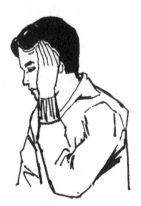

5. **Combing the Hair.** Separate the fingers and curve the hands slightly. Use them to comb the hair 24–50 times starting from the front hairline and moving backwards. Set the tongue against the palate and keep the breathing natural. Pay attention to the sensation under the palms.

6. **Sweeping the Gallbladder Channel.** Put the four fingers close together and curve them slightly. Scrape with the fingertips along the Gallbladder Channel

Figure 11

from above the ears backward via the frontal angle toward the back of the head (Fig. 11). Pay attention to the sensation under the palms. Respiration should be even and long. Scrape 5–10 times during expiration and stop scraping during inspiration. Do the exercise for 5–10 respiratory cycles.

7. **Rubbing the Back of the Head.** Clasp the hands against the lower part of the occipital bone (bone in the back, lower part of the skull) with the fingers interlocked. Rub the back of the head from the top downwards 5–10 times during expiration and stop rubbing during inspiration. Do this for 5–10 respiratory cycles, concentrating the mind on activities under the hands (Fig.12).

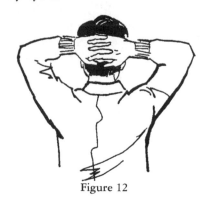

Figure 12

Application

Head and Face Exercise is suitable for invigorating the skin and preventing wrinkles in young people. It also treats hypertension, facial paralysis, headaches, dizziness, colds and migraines, and prevents and treats hair loss in older people. For grooming purposes, put the stress on the following three procedures: bathing the face, pushing the forehead, and combing the hair. Use natural respiration and pay attention to the sensation induced by the hand manipulation. Imagine that your wrinkles have vanished and the blood is circulating perfectly. Those with headaches and dizziness due to hypertension and neurosis should use the following: sweeping the gallbladder channel, massaging *Taiyang* (Extra 2), and scraping the back of the head. Pay attention to the sensation under the hands. Try to get the functional activities of Qi to move downwards during expiration in coordination with hand manipulation. Stop the manipulation during inspiration. Avoid respiratory suppression and violent rubbing or scraping.

Points for Attention

Practice the exercise 1–4 times a day. The number of hand manipulations and the force used should be increased gradually depending on the actual conditions of the individual. Avoid bursts of anger or mental stress. Lead a balanced life. If you feel dizzy or uncomfortable after mental work, do the exercise one or two times to dispel fatigue.

3.5 Eye Exercise *(Yan Gong)*

Functions: Regulates the blood of the Liver Channel, soothes the liver, and improves vision.

Methods

1. **Preparation**: Sit or stand, relax, look straight ahead, and expel any distracting thoughts.

2. **Moving the Eyeballs in an Infinity Pattern.** Move the eyeballs and imagine that there is a flow of Qi inside their orbits. Start the eye movements from slightly above the inner corner (the acupuncture point *Jingming* (U.B. 1)) of the left eye.

   Move the eyeballs along the upper side left orbit toward the outer corner (canthus) and then, along the lower side of the left orbit to the point *Jingming* (U.B. 1) of the right eye. Continue by moving the eyeballs along the upper side of the right orbit to the right outer corner (canthus), then along the lower side of the right orbit back to left *Jingming* (U.B. 1). In other words,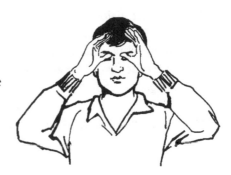

   Figure 13

   move the eyes in a figure-eight pattern. Do the exercise 8 times. Then repeat for another 8 times in the opposite direction starting from the right *Jingming* (U.B. 1). Breathe naturally during the exercise. Direct the flow of Qi by will and allow the mind to follow the movement of Qi.

3. **Pressing the Eyes to Guide Qi.** Use the thumbs to press the internal upper corners of the orbits and concentrate on this location. Press backward on the orbits while inhaling then gently press the eyeballs while exhaling so that a distending sensation in the eyes is produced. Do this 8 times (Fig. 13).

4. **Bathing the Eyes.** Close the eyes slightly. Rub the flats of the four fingers together until they are warm, and then rub the eyes from the inner corners to the outer corners 24 times (Fig. 14). Use natural respiration and focus the attention under the hands.

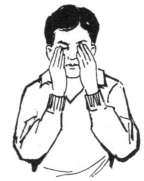

Figure 14

Application

This exercise is practiced to keep the eyes healthy as well as to prevent and cure near- and far-sightedness and astigmatism in adolescence. It also functions to regulate blood and Qi circulation in the Liver Channel in order to soothe the liver and improve eyesight. Better results can be obtained when it is done in combination with the exercise Soothing the Liver to Improve the Acuity of Vision. Eye Exercise can also be practiced for dizziness, discomfort of the eye, eye congestion, swelling, pain, and fatigue of the eye muscles in older people. At completion of the exercise, one should close the eyes slightly and rest for a moment.

Points for Attention

Practice the exercise 1–4 times a day. To relieve eye strain caused by reading or writing, practice methods 1 and 3 to allay eye fatigue and protect eyesight. Do not read in dim light and wear proper spectacles. Pay attention to eye hygiene and avoid eye fatigue.

3.6 Nose and Teeth Exercise *(Bichi Gong)*

Functions: Clears the nasal passages, prevents cavities by reinforcing the teeth.

Methods

1. **Preparation.** Assume a sitting or standing posture. Get rid of nasal discharge and become relaxed and quiet. Breathe naturally.

2. **Bathing the Nose.** Rub the dorsal (back) sides of the thumbs against each other until they are hot. Use them to rub the sides of the nose gently up and down. Rub the nose 5 times during each inspiration and expiration. Perform 6 respiratory cycles (Fig. 15).

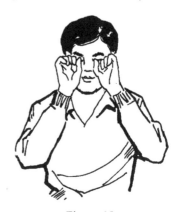

Figure 15

3. **Kneading the Nose Apex.** Put the tip of the middle finger of the right hand on the apex (tip) of the nose and knead it counterclockwise during inspiration and clockwise during expiration for 5 times each. Do this for 6 respiratory cycles.

4. **Tapping and Clenching the Teeth.** Tap the upper and lower teeth together 36 times and swallow the saliva that accumulates from this activity. Always clench the teeth during defeca-

tion or urination, and relax them gradually when finished. Breathe naturally and concentrate the mind on the teeth so as to consolidate vital essence.

Application

The Nose and Teeth Exercise can clear the nasal passages, strengthen the teeth, and prevent cavities. Long-term practice will yield sure benefits. This exercise is not only used for health preservation, but also for prevention and treatment of a stuffy nose, a runny nose with turbid discharge, a cold, and a toothache.

Points for Attention

Practice the exercise 1–2 times a day. For prevention and treatment of rhinitis, bathing the nose is the method of choice and should be practiced 2–4 times a day. Hand manipulation should be gentle and penetrating. To avoid skin injury, rough force should not be used. Pay attention to oral hygiene and expel any nasal discharge before practice.

3.7 Ear Exercise (Er Gong)

Functions: Prevents and treats ear trouble, dredges the channels, and improves hearing.

Methods

1. **Preparation.** Sit or stand in a relaxed manner. Use Inward-hearing and close the mouth and eyes. Breathe naturally and get rid of distracting thoughts.

2. **Striking the Heavenly Drum (Ming Tian Gu).** Using the palms of the hands, press the ears with the point *Laogong* (P 8) (located on the palms) aimed at the ear orifices. Resting the fingers on the back of the head. Cross the index fingers above the middle fingers and snap them to tap the back of the head lightly 24 times. You can hear drumming sound when doing this.

3. **Pressing the Ears to Guide Qi.** Press the ear orifices tightly with the palms so as to compress the inner ears and release them 10 times. Be sure to avoid forceful and violent pressing or releasing. Though the pressing should be tight and the release rapid, it must be done gently and moderately.

4. **Massaging the Auricles.** Pinch the top of the auricles (external portion of the ear) of the ear gently with the thumbs and the index fingers and massage from the top downwards at least 24 times until they are warm.

Application

This exercise is recommended for improving hearing, health preservation, and prevention and treatment of ear disorders. For treatment of tinnitus, deafness and earache, practice this exercise in combination with kidney replenishing exercises such as Taking Black Qi, Rubbing the Renal Region, or Rubbing *Yongquan* (K 1).

Points for Attention

Practice this exercise 1–2 times daily for health preservation, and 2–4 daily times for treatment of ear diseases. Do not exert too much force, especially when releasing the palms from the ears. Pay attention to ear hygiene, and keep constant Inward-hearing for inner cultivation. If you have tinnitus, rub the ear regions gently with the two palms and move the head slightly before doing the exercise.

3.8 Neck Exercise *(Jingxiang Gong)*

Functions: Prevents and cures neck troubles, activates the flow of blood in the channels and collaterals, and lubricates the joints.

Methods

1. **Preparation.** Assume a standing or sitting posture. Relax the neck, breathe naturally, and look straight ahead.

2. **Dredging *Fengchi*.** Knead the point *Fengchi* (G.B. 20) gently with the thumbs 10 times during each respiratory cycle for 14 cycles. Then with the thumb, index, and middle fingers clenched together like a beak, gently tap on *Fengchi* (G.B. 20) 30 times.

3. **Massaging *Tianzhu*.** Bend the head slightly forward. Rub the back of the neck, along its midline, with the fingertips of the four fingers on each hand from the top of the neck downwards 7 times during expiration. Stop rubbing during inspiration. Do this procedure for 8 respiratory cycles (Fig. 16).

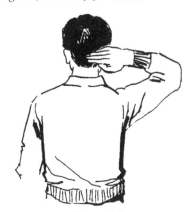

Figure 16

4. **Massaging the Blood Waves (*Xue Lang*).** Close the four fingers of the right hand and rub the right side of the neck near the carotid artery (blood wave region.) During expiration, rub (the left side first for men and the right side first for women) from under the jaw along the sternocleidomastoid muscle down to the clavicle. Stop rubbing during inspiration. Do this for 14 respiratory cycles (Fig.17). Change hands and rub the other side of the neck.

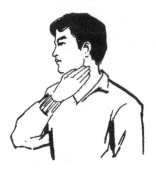

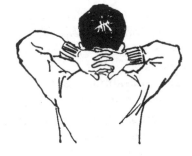

Figure 17   Figure 18

5. Turning the Neck to Guide Qi. Inhale while facing forward. Exhale and turn the head to the left. Inhale while returning to original position. Do this 8 times. Change directions and repeat another 8 times.

6. Pulling the Neck. Interlock the fingers of both hands to hold the back of the neck and pull the neck forwards during inspiration. At the same time, thrust the head backward and look upward at the same time. Relax during expiration. Do this for nine respiratory cycles (Fig. 18).

Application

This exercise is suitable for health preservation and for alleviating neck pain, cervical spondylopathy, stiff neck and fibrositis of the neck muscles. To treat hypertension, headache, dizziness or vertigo, methods 2 and 4 should be employed in combination with methods 5 and 6 of the Head and Face Exercise and with Psychosomatic Relaxation Exercise. For treatment of conditions such as cervical spondylophathy and stiffneck, methods 3, 5, and 6 are recommended.

Points for Attention

Practice the exercise 1–4 times a day. Try to practice it at least once each morning. The force exerted must be coordinated with the movements. The sphere of movements and the strength used should be increased gradually. The speed should be controlled and coordinated with breathing. Avoid resting the head on high pillows or bending the head over work for too long. Those who have to take such a position in their work should choose several methods from this exercise to keep the muscles and tendons relaxed, activate the blood in the channels and collaterals, lubricate the joints, and relieve fatigue.

3.9 Shoulder Arm Exercise (*Jianhi Gong*)

Functions: Prevents and treats disorders of the shoulders and arms, facilitates circulation of the blood in the Three Yang and Three Yin Channels of the hand, reduces swelling, allays pain, and lubricates the joints.

Methods

1. **Preparation.** Assume either standing or sitting posture, remove any distractions, relax, and breathe naturally.

2. **Pounding the Shoulders and Arms.** Make the left hand into a hollow fist and pound the external, internal, and anterior sides of the right arm from the shoulder to the wrist. Repeat this procedure for the left arm.

3. **Dredging the Three *Yin* and Three *Yang* Channels of Hand.** Sit erect and place the right hand on the right thigh with palm up. With the left palm, massage the internal side of the right arm from the uppermost aspect, along the Three *Yin* Channels of Hand down to the palm (Fig. 19). Exhale slowly and allow the mind to follow the massaging hand. Then turn the right hand, so the palm is down, and massage with the left palm from the back of the right palm along the Three *Yang* Channels of Hand up to the shoulder while inhaling and following the hand manipulation with the mind (Fig. 20). Practice this procedure 7 times then massage the point *Hegu* (L.I. 4) 36 times with the left hand. Avoid holding the breath during the exercise and relax the arms as much as possible. Dredge the Three *Yin* and Three *Yang* Channels of the Hand of the left arm in the same way, remembering to massage the point *Hegu* (L.I. 4) with the right hand.

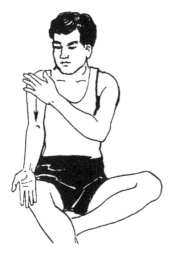

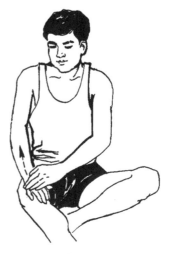

Figure 19   Figure 20

4. **Kneading *Quchi*.** Knead the point *Quchi* (L.I. 11) on the right arm with the left thumb 36 times. Do the same to the left *Quchi* (L.I. 11) with the right thumb.

5. ***Hegu*.** Knead the right and left *Hegu* (L.I. 4), with the left and right thumbs respectively, 36 times each.

Application

This exercise promotes the flow of Qi and blood in the Three *Yin* and *Yang* Channels of Hands, relieves swelling and pain, and lubricates the joints. It is recommended for conditions such as aching, pain, and numbness of the arm and shoulder, and sprains and weakness of the limbs. To treat arm and shoulder pain, do this exercise together with other methods such as flexing, stretching and rotating the shoulders, elbows and wrists.

Points for Attention

Practice this exercise once or twice a day. It can also be done following other exercises to regulate the Qi in the arms. Do not wash the hands or take a bath with cold water immediately after the exercise.

3.10 Chest Hypochondrium Exercise *(Xiongxie Gong)*

Functions: Treats disorders of the chest and hypochondrium (area of the abdomen beneath the lower ribs), relieves stuffiness of the chest, regulates and soothes the liver, relieves cough and reduces sputum.

Methods

1. **Preparation.** Stand or sit, breathe evenly, and relax.

2. **Pushing and Regulating *Tanzhong*.** Perform pushing massage with the index, middle, ring and small fingers, from the suprasternal notch (the notch at the top of the sternum) down to the xiphoid process 36 times. The fingers should point up while the hand moves down. Breathe naturally, and concentrate the mind on the activities under the fingers.

3. **Pushing the Chest to Regulate Qi.** With the right palm, perform pushing massage starting from the middle line of the chest outward to the left 5–10 times during expiration. Do not push during inspiration. Repeat this procedure for 10 respiratory cycles. With the left palm, massage the chest from the middle line outward to the right. The mind should follow the hand manipulations.

4. **Rubbing the Hypochondrium to Descend Qi.** This is done during expiration with the two palms doing pushing massage from the armpit to the sides of the abdomen. The left hand should be on the left, the right on the right.

Application

This exercise relieves chest stuffiness, regulates the flow of Qi, disperses liver depression, descends the deranged Qi, and reduces cough and sputum. It is indicated for chest pain, breathing disorders, profuse expectoration, dyspnea. For the treatment of asthma and bronchitis, it is advisable to do this exercise in combination with Lung Regulating Exercise or the method of uttering "Si."

Points for Attention

Practice the exercise once or twice a day. It can also be done following other Qigong exercising methods or as a closing or auxiliary practice. Be sure to keep fine, slow, even, and natural breathing during practice. Never forcefully hold the breath. Keep the muscles relaxed. This exercise should be practiced in an area that has fresh air, and the three steps of the exercise must be practiced in order.

3.11 Abdominal Exercise *(Fubu Gong)*

Functions: Prevents and treats disorders of the digestive system, strengthens the spleen, replenishes and regulates the stomach, invigorates the middle Jiao.

Methods

1. **Preparation.** Lie supine, relax the whole body, apply tongue against palate, and breathe naturally.

2. **Kneading the Abdomen to Reinforce Qi.** Place the right hand to the area of the point *Zhongwan* (Ren 12), and move it clockwise in circles to knead the abdomen 36 times. Then, place the same hand on the navel region, and move it first in clockwise and then counterclockwise circles 36 times each.

3. **Pushing the Abdomen to Promote Digestion.** Use a pushing massage on the abdomen with the four fingers or palms of the two hands. Start from the xiphoid process and move along the abdominal midline to the pubic symphysis 36 times. Then use the same technique starting again from the xiphoid process, separating the hands and pushing them obliquely downward 36 times. Carry out the manipulation during expiration and try to feel the sensation of Qi caused by the hand movement.

4. **Kneading the Abdomen to Strengthen Qi.** Place the right hand over the left and use them to knead the midpoint of the lower abdomen 36 times, then close the fingers, so that they look like a beak, and tap the midpoint with the fingertips 50–100 times.

Application

This exercise is suitable for general health. It is also used in the prevention and treatment of abdominal pain and distention, diarrhea, constipation, anorexia, colitis, gastritis, gastric and duodenal ulcers, and other disorders of the digestive system. For treatment of diarrhea and constipation, Abdominal Exercise can be practiced following Circulation Exercise to get better therapeutic effects. For treatment of ulcers or colitis, it is desirable to precede the exercise with Inner Health Cultivation Exercise or Health Promotion Exercise.

Points for Attention

Practice this exercise 1–2 times a day for preservation of health and 2–4 times for curing illness. Relieve bowels before practice. This exercise is should be practiced one hour after eating when you are neither full nor hungry. Hand manipulation should be coordinated with respiration and mental activities. Use proper speed and moderate strength. Never exert rough pressure.

3.12 Waist Exercise (Yaobu Gong)

Functions: Improves circulation in the lumbar region, strengthens the muscles and bones, reinforces the loins, and replenishes the kidneys.

Methods

1. **Preparation.** Stand erect with feet shoulder-width apart, relax, and breathe naturally.

2. **Moving the Waist to Strengthen the Muscles.** Stand with hands on the waist, and move the waist clockwise and counterclockwise 36 times in each direction (Fig.21).

3. **Pounding the Waist.** Turn hands into hollow fists and pound them against renal regions and the lumbosacral area 36 times each.

4. **Rubbing the Waist.** Rub the two palms against each other until they are hot, and then use them to rub the entire lumbar and renal regions until the regions are warm.

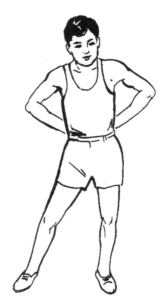

Figure 21

33

Application

This exercise is usually practiced for health preservation and the prevention and treatment of lumbago, soreness in the waist and weakness of the knees. Those with lower back pain due to lowered kidney function usually do this exercise in combination with such exercises as Nourishing the Kidney for Rejuvenation.

Points for Attention

Practice this exercise once or twice a day. Limit the frequency of sexual intercourse. The exercise can be done after practicing other exercises to enhance the effect of waist training.

3.13 Exercise of the Lower Limbs (Xiazhi Gong)

Functions: Strengthens the waist and legs, prevents and cures diseases of the lower limbs, relaxes the muscles and tendons, and activates the flow of blood in the channels and collaterals.

Methods

1. **Preparation.** Assume a sitting posture.

2. **Patting the Lower Limbs.** Slightly bend one leg and extend the other. Keep the hands stretched naturally, and use the palm to gently pat the stretched leg from the uppermost of the thigh down to the ankle 3–5 times. Do the same for other leg.

3. **Dredging the Three *Yin* and Three *Yang* Channels of the Foot.** Sit on something soft and assume the previous position. Place both hands on the exterior aspect of the leg where it connects to the waist. Conduct pushing massage along the Three *Yang* Channels of the Foot downward to the toes while exhaling and allow the mind to follow the hand manipulations (Fig.22). Then move the palms to the internal side of the foot and conduct pushing massage along the Three *Yin* Channels of the Foot up to the top of the thigh while inhaling. Allow the mind to follow the hand manipulations (Fig. 23). Repeat this method 7–9 times.

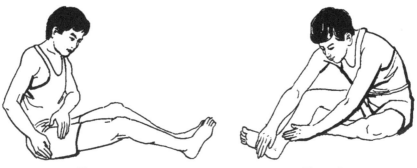

Figure 22   Figure 23

Application

This exercise functions to activate Qi and blood circulation in the Three *Yin* and Three *Yang* Channels of the Foot, strengthen the waist and legs, and expel wind and cold. It is also used for health preservation and prevention and treatment of sciatica and arthritis. It is also used to prevent and treat pain in the loins and knees caused by cold-dampness, for weakness and numbness of the lower limbs, and for relieving fatigue. The exercise can be done in combination with The Crane Village Qigong *(Hexiangzhuang Qigong)* or Simultaneous Moving Qigong *(Zifa Gong)*.

Points for Attention

To preserve health, practice this exercise 1–2 times a day. To prevent and treat disease, it should be practiced 2–4 times a day. This exercise can be practiced when you feel tired to relieve fatigue. It is advisable to wear shorts during this exercise.

3.14 Heart Regulation Exercise *(Lixin Gong)*

Functions: Regulates the Qi and blood of the Heart channel, invigorates the heart, relaxes the mind, promotes blood circulation, and dredges the channels.

Methods

1. **Taking Red Qi.** Assume the standing, sitting or lying posture and breathe naturally. Remove any distractions. Tap the upper and lower teeth together 36 times and use the tongue to stir the resulting saliva. Swallow the saliva 3 times, after the tapping is finished, and send it mentally down to the point *Zhongwan* (Ren 12) (the middle part of the gastric cavity). Imagine that there is red in front of your face. Inhale the red nasally and fill the mouth with it. Send the red slowly down to the heart during expiration to coordinate the heart and kidney. The coordination between all the channels in the body will naturally follow. Do this 7–14 times. Resume starting posture to complete exercise.

2. **Rubbing the Chest and "Ha."** Prepare as mentioned above, tap the teeth, and swallow the saliva. As soon as the saliva is swallowed, put the right palm above the heart and inhale slowly. Then exhale slowly while pronouncing "Ha" and concentrating the mind on the activities beneath the hand, which should move gently in a clockwise direction (Fig. 24). Practice this for 6–12 respiratory cycles.

3. **Invigorating the Heart and Guiding Qi.** Assume the standing or sitting posture, relax the body all over, and breathe naturally. Stick the tongue against the palate and gently put

the two palms against each other in front of the chest (Fig. 25). Keep still for a moment while concentrating the mind on the *Diantian*. Turn the palms so they face outward and stretch the arms to the back along the sides of the body and (Fig. 26) keep still for a moment. Then turn the palms upwards and pull them beside the chest (Fig. 27). Stretch the hands slowly forward with force focused on the tips of the middle fingers (Fig.28). Rotate the palms out-

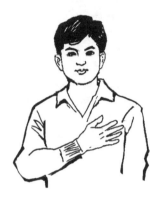

Figure 24

ward with a little force on the thenar eminence major (the base of the thumb). Next clench the fists as if dragging something heavy, and pull towards the back keeping the fists along the sides of the body (Fig.29). Lift the right hand—as if holding something heavy—up to the chest, turn the palm outward, and push it forward (Fig.30). Pull back the right hand and repeat this procedure with the left hand. To end the exercise, return to the starting posture. Repeat these procedures 2–3 times each.

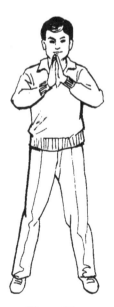

Figure 25

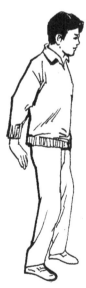

Figure 26

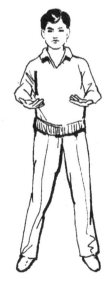

Figure 27

Application

This exercise is recommended in the prevention and treatment of syndromes manifested by common or severe palpitation, pain and insomnia as seen in coronary heart disease, hypertension, arrhythmia, rheumatic heart disease, and cardiac neurosis. Those who are feeble may practice this exercise in the sitting or lying posture. Those with deficiency syndromes should practice Taking Red Qi, which has the effect of invigorating the heart, nourishing the blood, and calming the mind. This method can also be carried out in combination with Invigorating the Heart and Guiding Qi to activate the flow of Qi and blood through the channels and collaterals. Those with heart failure should emphasize heart maintenance and do the exercise in combination with Inner Health Cultivation Exercise concentrating the mind only on the *Dantian*.

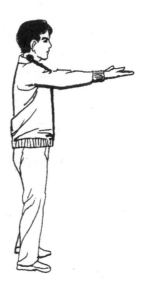

Figure 28

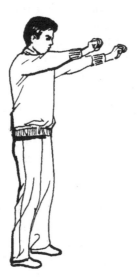

Figure 29

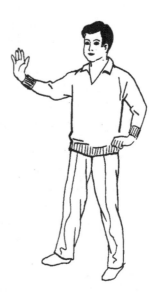

Figure 30

Those with excess syndrome should use Rubbing the Chest and "Ha" which emphasizes the purging pathogenic factors and the removal of stasis. To promote the flow of Qi along the Heart Channel, practice Rubbing the Chest and "Ha" in combination with Invigorating the Heart and Guiding Qi. For the purpose of health preservation, use Rubbing the Chest and "Ha" as the chief method.

Points for Attention

Practice this exercise facing south, 1–3 times daily. Keep yourself lighthearted, lead a regular life, and eat a moderate diet. This exercise should be practiced in a quiet place to avoid fright. The duration and the frequency of exercise are decided according to the health status of the individual. The general principle is to have a sense of well-being and be free from fatigue after the exercise is finished.

3.15 Spleen Regulation Exercise *(Lipi Gong)*

Functions: Regulates the blood of the Spleen Channel, strengthens the spleen to replenish Qi, and regulates the stomach to promote digestion.

Methods

1. **Taking Yellow Qi.** Assume a standing or sitting posture, and relax the body all over. Breathe naturally, and expel any distracting thoughts. Tap the upper and lower teeth together 36 times, and stir the resulting saliva with the tongue. Swallow the saliva three times after the tapping, and imagine that you are sending it down to the point *Zhongwan* (Ren 12) (the middle part of the gastric cavity). Imagine that there is yellow in front of your face. Breathe in the yellow, and fill your mouth with it. During expiration, send it slowly down to *Zhongwan* (Ren 12) and then disperse it to the extremities, skin, and hair. Repeat this procedure 5–10 times. Resume starting posture to complete exercise.

2. **Rubbing Zhongwan Area and "Hu."** Assume a standing or sitting posture. Place the right palm gently against the upper abdomen *Zhongwan* (Ren 12) and exhale slowly. During expiration, rub the upper abdomen in a clockwise direction with the right palm (Fig. 31) and utter "Hu" at the same time. Do this for 10–20 respiratory cycles.

3. **Dredging the Spleen and Stomach.** Assume the standing posture, relax, and breathe naturally. Swing the arms left and right using the waist as the axle (Fig. 32), allow the eyesight to follow the same direction of the swinging arms, and concentrate the mind on the heels. Next sit on heels, rest the palms

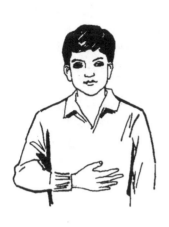

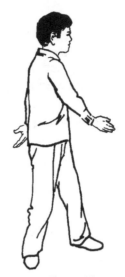

Figure 31   Figure 32

on the head and remain quiet for a while. Prostrate the upper part of the body with the hips raised and look back over the left shoulder like a tiger eyeing the distance (Fig. 33). Then turn the head and look over the right shoulder in the same fashion. Repeat the procedures 5 times.

Application

This exercise is beneficial to health preservation and prevention of abdominal distention, diarrhea, and constipation. It is indicated for chronic gastritis, duodenal ulcer, colitis, and gastric and intestinal neurosis. For increased effects this exercise can be practiced in combination with Abdominal Exercise. It is preferable, that patients with hypo-function of the spleen and cold stomach conditions practice Taking Yellow Qi, which has the function of strengthening the spleen and replenishing Qi. Those with excess heat syndromes should practice Rubbing Zhongwan and "Hu," which promotes digestion by invigorating the stomach and eliminating pathogenic factors. Patients with syndromes of either deficiency or excess type can practice Dredging the Spleen and Stomach as well as Inner Health Cultivation Exercise.

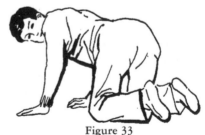

Figure 33

Points for Attention

Practice this exercise 1–4 times a day. Lead a normal life. Do not eat or drink too much at one meal. Avoid doing the exercise when you are too full or too hungry. This exercise should not be practiced by those with bleeding and perforation in the stomach or duodenum.

3.16 Lung Regulation Exercise *(Lifei Gong)*

Functions: Regulates the Qi and blood of the Lung Channel, replenishes the lung, promotes the dispersing function of the lung, sends down abnormally ascending Qi, relieves cough and resolves phlegm.

Methods

1. **Taking White Qi.** Assume a standing, sitting or lying posture, relax, breathe naturally, and dispel any distractions. Tap the upper and lower teeth together 36 times, and stir the resulting saliva with the tongue. Swallow the saliva in three segments after the tapping, and imagine sending it first to the chest and then to the *Dantian.* Imagine that there is white in front of the face. Inhale the white and fill the mouth with it. During expiration, send it slowly down to the lungs, then to the *Dantian*, and to the skin and hair of the whole body. Do this 9 or 18 times. Resume starting posture to complete exercise.

2. **Rubbing the Chest and "Si."** Assume a standing or sitting posture. Place the palms flat on each side of the chest. Inhale slowly. Say "Si" during expiration, and rub the chest with both hands in a circular manner (Fig.34). Repeat the procedures for 6–12 respiratory cycles.

3. **Regulating the Lung and Guiding Qi.** Sit cross-legged, breathe naturally, and press the palms against the ground at the sides of the body. Square the chest to get a deep inspiration. Hold the breath for a second (Fig. 35), then arch the back and pull in the chest, and expire simultaneously (Fig. 36). Do this 4–9 times.

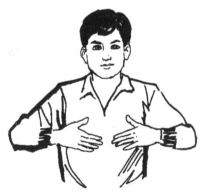

Figure 34

40

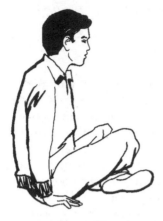

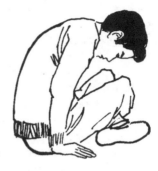

Figure 35   Figure 36

4. Regulating the Lung with Knee Movement. Stand with
legs close together, put the palms on both kneecaps, and slowly
rub the knee joints clockwise and counterclockwise four times
in each direction (Fig. 37). Inhale when rubbing the knees
counterclockwise and exhale when rubbing clockwise.

Application

This exercise is suitable for keeping the
lungs healthy and for the prevention and
treatment of chest stuffiness, chest pain,
shortness of breath, and profuse expectoration. It is also indicated for chronic bronchitis, pulmonary emphysema, and bronchial
asthma. The exercise Taking White Qi
invigorates the lungs and is effective for
deficiency syndromes. The exercise Rubbing
The Chest and "Si" is effective for excess
syndromes. The Lung Regulation exercise
will be more effective if it is done in combination with the Chest Exercise.

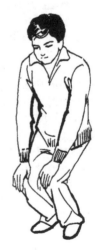

Points for Attention

Practice this exercise 2–4 times a day,
10–40 minutes each time. Smoking, drink-

Figure 37

ing, and consuming raw, cold, or irritating food should be avoided
during practice. For people with mild lung problems practicing in the
park or woods where the air is fresh is recommended. Those with
infection of the lung should lie on the diseased side when resting. If you
cannot hold back coughing during practice, stop the movement to
cough up the phlegm, and then continue the exercise.

3.17 Liver Regulation Exercise *(Ligan Gong)*

Functions: Regulates the Qi and blood of the Liver channel, soothes the liver, and subdues hyperactivity of the liver.

Methods

1. **Taking Green Qi.** Assume a standing, sitting or lying posture, relax, breathe naturally, and expel the distractions. Place the tip of the tongue on the palate. Tap the upper and lower teeth together 36 times, and stir the resulting saliva with the tongue. After tapping, swallow the saliva in three segments sending each one down to the hypochondria and further to the *Dantian*. Imagine green and inhale it through the nose to the mouth. Send it slowly down during expiration to the hypochondria and then to the *Dantian*. Repeat 8 or 16 times. Resume starting posture to complete exercise.

2. **Rubbing the Hypochondrium and "Xu."** Assume the standing or sitting posture. Place the palms against the ribs and inhale slowly. Say "Xu" during exhalation with the palms rubbing about the ribs (Fig. 38). Practice the exercise for 10–20 respiratory cycles.

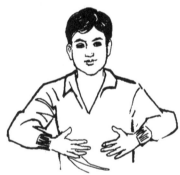

Figure 38

3. **Soothing the Liver and Guiding Qi.** Stand relaxed and quiet with the arms falling naturally at the sides, the palms facing downward. Pull the five fingers slightly upward, and press the palms downward with a little force. Imagine that Qi has been directed to the center of the palms and further to the fingertips. Lift and press the palms downwards three times (Fig. 39), inhaling on the lift and exhaling when pressing down. Next lift the two hands up to the chest with palms facing away from the body (Fig. 40). Concentrate the mind on the palms and push them outwards during exhalation; pull them back during inspiration. Next, stretch both hands towards the respective side like birds stretching their wings, with the fingers tilted upward (Fig. 41). Guide Qi to the center of the palms and further to the fingertips. Bend the elbows to bring the hands in during inhalation, and press them back out during expiration. Do this three times. When the last movement is completed, pull the palms back naturally to the chest, palms upward and fingertips

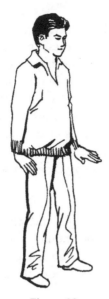

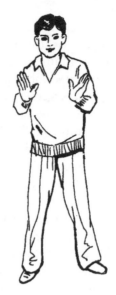

Figure 39   Figure 40

pointing at each other. Concentrate the mind on the two palms and then turn them to face downward (Fig. 42). Push the palms downward to the pubic symphysis, directing Qi to the lower *Dantian*. Turn the palms upward to hold Qi and raise it up to the Middle *Dantian* (*Tanzhong* (Ren 17)). Carry out the procedures three times, then drop the hands to the sides of the body to end the exercise.

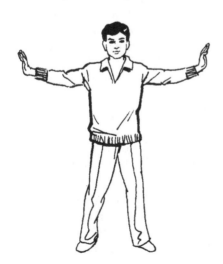

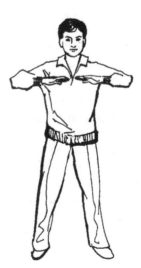

Figure 41   Figure 42

Application

Liver Regulation Exercise is used for health preservation and for the prevention and treatment of dizziness, vertigo, bitterness in the mouth, dry throat, and fullness and stuffiness in the chest and hypochondrium. It is also indicated for hypertension, neurosis, chronic hepatitis, cholecystitis, and enlargement of the liver and spleen. For liver and gallbladder syndromes of the excess type, it is recommended to use Rubbing the Hypochondrium and "Xu." For deficiency syndromes of the gallbladder and liver, practice Taking Green Qi. For treatment of both types of syndromes, practice Liver Regulation Exercise in combination with Soothing the Liver and Guiding Qi.

Points for Attention

Practice this exercise 1–4 times a day. Avoid anger and keep a light heart during the exercise. Those with hypertension should do the exercise in combination with Psychosomatic Relaxation Exercise, Sweeping the Gallbladder Channel from exercise 3.4, and Massaging the Blood Wave from exercise 3.8.

3.18 Kidney Regulation Exercise *(Lishen Gong)*

Functions: Regulates the blood and of the Kidney Channel, nourishes the kidneys, strengthens Yang (vital function), and invigorates primordial energy.
Methods

1. **Taking Black Qi.** Assume a standing, sitting, or lying posture and relax. Place the tongue against the palate and expel distractions. Tap the upper and lower teeth together 36 times, and stir the resulting saliva with the tongue. After tapping, swallow the saliva in three segments sending each one down to the *Dantian*. Imagine the color black. Inhale it nasally and fill the mouth with it. Send it slowly to the kidneys during expiration. Repeat this 6–12 times. Resume starting posture to complete exercise.

2. **Rubbing the Abdomen and "Chui."** Stand or sit, place one hand against the lower abdomen, and inhale slowly. Utter "Chui" when exhaling and stroke the lower abdomen with the palm simultaneously. (Fig.43) Repeat this for 10 or 20 respiratory cycles.

3. **Strengthening the Kidney and Guiding Qi.** Stand erect, make hollow fists and apply them against the soft parts at the sides of the waist (the kidney area). Turn the waist counterclockwise and clockwise (Fig. 44) for 6 times in each direction.

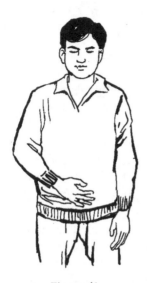

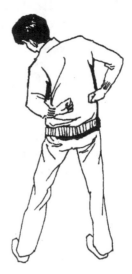

Figure 43   Figure 44

4. Rubbing the Renal Regions. Stand or sit, put the two hands on the sides of the waist, and then rub the entire area 36 times while concentrating the mind on the waist.

Application

The Kidney Regulation Exercise is used for health preservation and for the prevention and treatment of pain along the spinal column, tinnitus, deafness, frequent urination, aversion to cold, and coldness or dampness of the genitals. It is also used to treat nephritis, neurosis, and cystitis. Those with kidney deficiency may practice Taking Black Qi. Rubbing the Abdomen and "Chui" may be practiced by those with dampness and itching of the genitals due to dampness and heat of the lower *Jiao* (*Xiajiao* lower portion of the body cavity). The exercise can be performed with emphasis on Strengthening the Kidney and Guiding Qi to treat syndromes of both deficiency and excess types. For the middle aged and older people, frequent practice of Rubbing the Kidney will help to invigorate *Yang* and strengthen the kidneys. Strengthening the Kidney and Guiding Qi and Rubbing the Kidney are also suitable for those with deficiency of Kidney *Yang* manifested by pain and weakness of the waist, spermatorrhea and impotence.

Points for Attention

Practice the exercise once in the morning and once in the evening or up to 4 times a day. Lead a balanced life with moderate sexual activity. Young people should avoid masturbation so as to cure seminal or involuntary emission.

3.19 Automatic Circulation Exercise *(Zhoutian Zizhuan Gong also Fu Lun Zi Zhuan, or Xing Ting)*

Functions: Increases circulation and mental activities.

Method

Sit or lie supine. Relax all over, breathe naturally, apply the tongue against the palate, and concentrate the mind on the navel. Concentrate on the navel as the center of a circle and imagine moving the abdominal muscles during inspiration. During inspiration imaging moving the abdominal muscles from the center point clockwise to a point above the navel. During this part of the movement one should silently say, "The white tiger is hiding in the east." During expiration continue the movement to complete the circle while silently saying, "The green dragon is hiding in the west." Continue this movement around the naval 36 times starting with a very small circle and gradually making it larger each time. The circles should expand from the navel until they cover the flanks and xiphoid process. Repeat this process in the opposite direction starting from the center point beneath the navel moving in a counterclockwise direction to the point opposite the starting point below the naval. During this part of the movement inhale and silently say, "The green dragon is hiding in the west." Complete the circle counterclockwise during expiration while saying, "The white tiger is hiding in the east." Practice the counterclockwise movement 36 times. Starting with a large circle and gradually make it smaller, returning to the starting point directly under the navel. Beginners may first try to direct Qi to rotate by means of respiration and movement of the abdominal muscles. As soon as they are skilled, they will be able to direct the intrinsic Qi to rotate around the navel by will alone. To complete this exercise, rub the abdomen clockwise and counterclockwise for 36 times in each direction.

Application

Automatic Circulation Exercise may be used for rehabilitation, general health care of the aged and middle-aged, and disease prevention. This exercise yields good therapeutic effects for diseases of the digestive system such as gastric and duodenal ulcer, gastritis, enteritis and hepatitis. To treat syndromes such as abdominal distention or pain, impairment by overeating, and constipation, practice the circle clockwise 81 times. For deficiency syndromes manifested by diarrhea, poor appetite and weakness of the limbs, practice the circle counterclockwise 81 times. Better results can be achieved if the exercise is practiced together with the Abdominal Exercise.

Points for Attention

Practice the exercise 2–4 times daily for health preservation and 4–6 times for treatment of diseases. This exercise can be practiced flexibly outside of regular practice hours. For example, it can be practiced after work or when the symptoms of a disease become severe, in which case it can be done until the symptoms improve. Persistent practice of this exercise should help regulate the *Yin* and *Yang* of the body. Keep yourself relaxed and comfortable during practice. Avoid forced holding of breath and mental strain. Be sure to defecate or urinate before doing the exercise. Any desire for defecation or urination may lead to diseases caused by mixing clear Qi with the turbid Qi. Keep a balanced diet. Overeating may cause stagnation of Qi while hunger may result in weakness of in motion.

3.20 Circulation Exercise *(Zhoutian Gong)*

This exercise is also known as Large Circulation of Qi *(Da Zhou Tian)*, Small Circulation of Qi *(Xiao Zhou Tian)*, and Exercise for Formation of Active Substance in the Body *(Nei Dan Shu)*. Only Small Circulation of Qi is described in this section.

Functions: Strengthens the immune and circulatory systems and preserves health.

Method

Sit cross-legged on a bed or upright on a stool. Pull in the chest and keep the spinal column straightened. Keep your neck straight (by picturing a light object on the head) and your shoulders relaxed. Close your eyes slightly and stick the tongue against the palate. Breathe evenly and concentrate the mind. Use abdominal respiration at first and then change to reverse breathing when you become familiar with the exercise. Respiration should be adjusted so that it is fine, gentle, soft, and long. Concentrate the mind vaguely on the *Dantian*. The movement of the abdominal muscles should be coordinated along with the breathing, which should feel lively and at ease. After a certain period of training, you may feel a kind of warmness in the *Dantian*, which will increase in intensity as you practice. When enough warmth has been accumulated, a flow of the hot Qi can be felt. With your mind, follow this energy from the along the *Du* Channel via the acupuncture point *Huiyin* (Ren 1) and the coccyx, upward to the vertex (top of the head) and cheeks, along the *Ren* Channel down to the chest and abdomen, and finally back to the starting point, the *Dantian*. This completes what is known as the small circulation. After the exercise, you should always concentrate the mind on the *Dantian* for a while to move Qi back to its origin. End the exercise by rubbing the hands and face.

Application

Circulation Exercise is used mainly for rehabilitation and health preservation. It is also taken as a basic exercise for treatment of chronic diseases.

Points for Attention

Practice Circulation Exercise 2–4 times a day, 10–60 minutes each time. Increase the frequency and duration of your practice based on your own condition. Before doing the exercise, loosen the waist belt, defecate completely and stay lighthearted. Never practice when you are too full or hungry. The effects of this exercise can only be achieved naturally. Do not force yourself to gain quick results.

3.21 Exercise for Soothing the Liver and Improving Acuity of Vision (Shugan Mingmu Gong)

Functions: Dredges the Liver Channel to nourish the liver, improves eyesight, relaxes the neck and back muscles, relieves muscular spasms of the eyes, and promotes recovery from fatigue.

Methods

1. **Preparation.** Stand relaxed and quiet, place the feet apart as wide as the shoulders, drop the hands naturally at the sides of the body, picture supporting an object on the head, pull in the chest and straighten the back, relax the loins and knees, look straight forward, and breathe naturally.

2. **Vision Regulation.** Look straight ahead and fix your eyes on a second point. Then, look farther and farther until you reach your limit and fix your eyes on a point. Stare at the point for a moment and then draw the vision gradually back to first point. Do this 4 times. Next look straight ahead, as far as possible, and simultaneously turn the eyeballs clockwise and counter-clockwise 4 times each. Breathe naturally during these procedures.

3. **Turning the Neck and Moving the Eyeballs.** Look into the distance, turn the neck clockwise and counterclockwise for 4 times each with the eyes following the movement of the neck. Inhale when the neck turns backwards and exhale when it turns for-wards (Fig. 45).

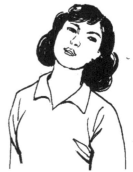

Figure 45

4. **Throwing Out the Chest and Relaxing the Back.** Raise the arms to the chest with the elbows bent and palms towards the breasts. Pull the elbows backward to throw out the chest and inspire at the same time. Relax the back and expire. Do this 8 times (Fig 46).

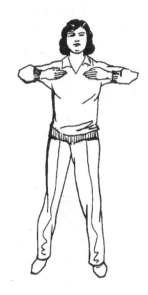

5. **Pressing Acupuncture Point *Jingming* and Guiding Qi.** Press the point *Jingming* (U.B. 1) with the thumbs while concentrating the mind on the eyes. Press toward the orbits and backward during inspiration. Then squeeze the eyeballs gently during expiration while saying "Xu" (Fig. 47). The proper pressing should produce a sensation of soreness and distention but not pain.

Figure 46

6. **Pressing the Acupuncture Point *Yuyao* and Guiding Qi.** Place the two thumbs on the point *Yuyao* (Extra 5) and concentrate the mind on the eyes. Press towards the orbits during inspiration and press the eyeballs gently during expiration while saying "Xu." Try to get the sensation of soreness and distention without pain.

7. **Pressing Acupuncture Point *Qiubou* and Guiding Qi.** Place the middle fingers on point *Qiubou* (Extra 7) and put the index finger lightly on the point *Sizhukong* (S.J. 23). Press the orbit backward with the middle fingers during inspiration, and squeeze the eyeballs gently during expiration while saying "Xu" (Fig. 48).

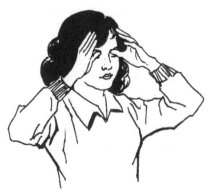

Figure 47

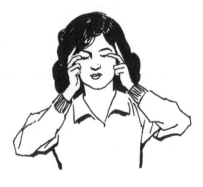

Figure 48

8. **Bathing the Eyes.** Use natural respiration. Place the four fingers of the left hand on the left eye and the four fingers of the right hand on the right eye, and rotate gently (the left hand clockwise and the right counterclockwise) 8 times then reverse (Fig. 49).

9. **Bathing the Face.** Place the palms on the cheeks and rotate and knead gently, in the same direction and for the same number of times as in the exercise "Bathing the Eyes." Use natural respiration (Fig. 50).

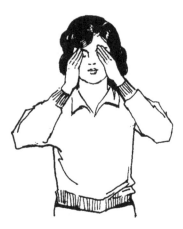

Figure 49

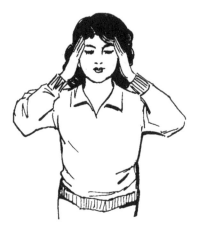

Figure 50

10. **Regulating Qi.** Close the eyes lightly, bend the elbows and raise the hands in front of the abdomen with palms facing upward (Fig. 51). Lift the palms slowly to the level of the eyes and rotate the palms slowly throughout the motion, so the palms end up the eyes. During this movement inspire and concentrate the mind on the eyes. Lift the two hands to almost the top of the head and then begin expiration. While still concentrating on the palms, lower the two hands to the level of the abdomen while continuing to exhale. Do this for 8 times before returning the hands to the starting posture to end the exercise.

Application

This exercise functions mainly in the prevention and treatment of myopia and astigmatism in adolescents and in the health care of eyes in the young and middle-aged. There should be no distracting thoughts while practicing this exercise. Mental activities and hand manipulations

should be coordinated closely. There may be
sensations like depressing and tugging
between the palms and the eyes, itching in
the eyelids, and warmth or coldness in the
eyes. These are normal effects of activities.

Points for Attention

Practice the exercise once in the morning
and once in the evening. Avoid overstrain of
the eyes. If you have to read for a long time,
do some of the above exercises to protect your
vision. Do not make the distance between
your eyes and the object too short, read in
dim light or while lying or standing.
Remember to look at a distant object regular-
ly. Stare at the object for a while and draw
back the sight slowly.

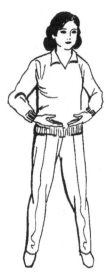

Figure 51

3.22 Exercise for Nourishing the Kidney for Rejuvenation *(Yangshen Huichun Gong)*

Functions: Dredges the channels, reinforces the kidneys, tonifies the Yang, and prolongs life.

This exercise is a superior Qigong *regime for nourishing the kidney and building up the health in the old and middle-aged.*

Methods

1. **Preparation.** Stand quietly with feet
   shoulder-width apart. Allow the hands
   to hang naturally, and keep the neck
   and spine straightened as if supporting
   an object on the head. Your knees
   should be relaxed and slightly bent,
   while the toes clutch the ground. Keep
   your tongue against the palate; your
   eyes should look ahead but see nothing.
   Breathe evenly, with the mind concentrated on the *Dantian*. Stand this way
   for 3–5 minutes (Fig. 52).

2. **Contracting the Anus and Guiding
   Qi.** Proceed from the last stance. Use
   reverse abdominal respiration. During
   inspiration, apply the tongue against
   the palate and shrink the neck, raising
   the shoulders slightly. Pull in the chest

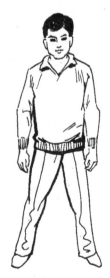

Figure 52

51

and abdomen and contract the anus, while lifting the heels slowly to stand on tiptoe and direct the Qi to circulate along the *Du* Channel up to the top of the head. During expiration, relax the anus, the abdomen, and then the whole body. Your heels should fall slowly onto the ground while directing the Qi along the *Ren* Channel down to the *Dantian*. Do this exercise 8 times. When directing Qi upwards, do not concentrate the mind too hard. Think that it is circulating correctly whether you feel it or not. Hypertensives may just think of the point *Yongquan* (K 1) without directing Qi to circulate upwards.

3. **Infinity Pattern Shoulder Movement.** Proceed from the last stance. Relax and breathe naturally. Turn the shoulders in an infinity pattern (figure-eight pattern) with the waist as the axle. Male practitioners should turn the left shoulder first and female should start with the right (Fig. 53). Turn the shoulders 8 times in each direction, according to the health status of the individual.

4. **Rounding the Crotch and Shaking the Body All Over.** Place the feet apart a little wider than shoulders-width, slightly contract the muscles of the legs with the knees pulling some-what toward each other to round the crotch (Fig. 54). Breathe naturally, close the eyes gently, and relax the jaw. Keep the lower abdomen in a state as if you were holding back defecating. Bend and straighten the knees alternately to lead the body to oscillate up and down. Gently click together the upper and lower teeth, while either vibrating the outer sexual organs, or closing and opening them freely. Do this for 5–30 minutes each time or for a desirable duration according to one's health status.

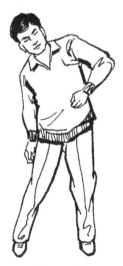

Figure 53

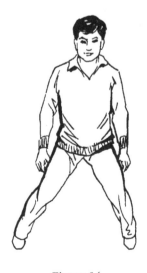

Figure 54

Application

With its satisfactory effects for strengthening the kidney *Yang* and reinforcing the vital essence, Exercise for Nourishing the Kidney for Rejuvenation is well suited for preserving the health of old and middle-aged people. It is also used to treat impotence, prospermia, listlessness, lassitude of the limbs, graying of hair, and premature senilism, hypomnesis and other syndromes. This exercise can be done in combination with Waist and/or Abdomen Exercise.

Points for Attention

For health preservation, practice the exercise once in the morning and once at night. Increase the frequency of practice if it is done to treat disease. Lead a regular life with a moderate sex life. Defecate before practice and dress in loosely fitted clothes. Be natural and quiet, and avoid negative thoughts.

3.23 Exercise of Taking Essence from the Sun and the Moon *(Cai Rijing Yuehua Gong)*

Functions: Balances Yin and Yang of the body, re-establishes a connection with nature.

Methods

1. **Taking Essence from the Sun.** Stand quiet and relaxed while facing the sun with the feet shoulder-width apart. Breathe evenly and expel distracting thoughts. When the sun rises from the horizon, close the eyes but not too tightly, so as to see the soft and reddish sunlight. Naturally inhale the sun's essence and imagine filling your mouth with it. Stop inhaling and relax the mind. During expiration, slowly swallow the sun's essence leading it down to the *Dantian*. Repeat the inhalation-swallowing cycle 9 times. Stay quiet and relaxed with the mind concentrated for a minute. Then move the body freely to end the exercise.

2. **Taking Essence from the Moon.** Select an open place with fresh air, and stand quiet and relaxed. Breathe naturally, expel distractions, and face the moon. Close the eyes to see only the faint light of the moon, and slowly inhale the moon's essence with both the mouth and nose. Imagine that the moon's essence is filling the mouth. Stop focusing on the breath, and concentrate your attention. During expiration, swallow the moon essence leading it down to the *Dantian*. Do this 6 times. Keep quiet for a minute then move the body freely for a while to end the exercise.

Application

The exercise Taking Essence from the Sun can treat intolerance of cold due to *Yang* insufficiency, coldness of the extremities, weakness of the spleen and stomach, and listlessness. Taking Essence from the Moon can treat hyperactivity of fire due to *Yin* deficiency; fever, thirst, and restlessness; feverish sensation in the palms and soles; and pain in the loins and knees. For general health, you should set the time and duration of the exercise flexibly according to your own schedule.

Points for Attention

For health preservation, practice the exercise Taking Essence from the Sun 3–7 times on the first, second and third day of a month of the lunar calendar. Perform Taking Essence from the Moon 3 times from the fifteenth to seventeenth day of a month of the lunar calendar. Those with insufficiency of *Yin* or *Yang* can do these exercises at other times besides the above mentioned dates. Do not do these exercises on cloudy, rainy or windy days. If the symptoms have subsided, then perform the exercise in the way defined for health preservation. Be sure to select an environment that has a supply of fresh air, be lighthearted and avoid anger.

3.24 Filth Elimination Exercise (Dihui Gong)

Functions: Eliminates intestinal pathogenic factors.

Method

Assume the sitting or lying postures. Relax and press the tongue against the palate. Close the eyes slightly, and breathe evenly. Imagine Qi whirling from left to right from the mouth to the stomach and carrying the genuine Qi to the large intestines, where it drives pathogenic factors from the intestines and out of the anus. Then inhale and contract the anus gently to close it. Conduct the genuine Qi whirling from right to left, upward through the intestine and out of the upper orifice of the stomach. Repeat this procedure 5–10 times. After the exercise, concentrate the mind on the *Diantian* for a moment to bring genuine Qi back to its origin. Rub the abdomen, hands, and face for a while to end the exercise.

Application

Filth Elimination Exercise is recommended for symptoms due to excess heat and the retention of damp-heat and waste in the intestines. This condition manifests as constipation, abdominal distention, nausea, vomiting, and fullness and discomfort in the epigastrium.

Points for Attention

Rub the abdomen clockwise 36 times before doing the exercise and counterclockwise for another 36 times after doing it. Practice this exercise 3 or 4 times a day. Increase the frequency if the symptoms are severe. As soon as the turbid Qi is driven out of the anus, reverse the mind to bring genuine Qi back. This exercise is **not suitable** for deficiency syndromes manifested as constipation due to *Yin* deficiency, prolapsed rectum, tenesmus, and distention of the anus due to Qi deficiency.

3.25 Daoyin Exercise for Ascending and Descending Yin and Yang *(Shengjiang Yin Yang Daoyin Gong)*

Functions: Regulates circulation within the Three Yin and Three Yang Channels of the Foot and Three Yin and Three Yang Channels of the Hand, establishing equilibrium of the Yin and Yang.

Method

Stand erect with feet shoulder-width apart and allow the hands to fall naturally at the sides of the body. Place the tongue against the palate with the eyes looking straight ahead and the neck straightened as if supporting an object on the head. The shoulders should be relaxed and the elbows dropped. Breathe evenly, and concentrate the mind on the *Dantian*. Slowly bend the waist forward allowing the hands to form natural fists and fall as low as possible in front of the feet. Simultaneously, direct Qi of the Three *Yang* Channels of the Foot from the head along the back, hips, and lower limbs to the feet. Next, straighten the waist slowly with fists clenched as if gripping something tightly. At the same time, direct the Qi of the Three *Yang* Channels of the Foot to flow to the acupuncture point *Yongquan* (K 1). Continue to direct Qi along the Three *Yin* Channels of the Foot up to the lower limbs, abdomen, and finally the chest. Continuing from the last movement, open the fists and turn them into palms facing upward, lift the palms forward and upward until the arms are directly in front of the body and slightly bent. Direct the Qi of the Three *Yin* Channels of the Foot up to the chest, along the Three *Yin* Channels of the Hand, to the upper limbs, and finally to the point Inner *Laogong* (P 8). Pull back the hands naturally to the chest, with the palms facing the chest and elbows out, directing Qi of the Three *Yang* Channels of the Hand to flow from Inner *Laogong* (P 8) to Outer *Laogong* (P 8), along the Three *Yang* Channels of the Hand, then upwards to the shoulders and head. Clench the hands and direct Qi of the Three *Yang* Channels of the Foot downward as you did in the beginning movement. Make the Qi flow this way for 36 repetitions. The movements should be integrated with breathing. Exhale when directing Qi of the Three *Yang* Channels of the Foot and the Three *Yin* Channels of the Hand downwards. Inhale when directing Qi of the of the Three *Yin* Channels of the Foot and the Three *Yang* Channels of the Hand upwards. Mental activities should follow the circulation of the Qi in the channels.

Application

This *Daoyin* exercise can regulate Qi in all of the Twelve Channels, promote good health, and aid in the recovery process from chronic diseases.

Points for Attention

Practice this exercise 1–4 times a day. It can be practiced before doing dynamic or static Qigong, by itself, or in combination with *Daoyin* Exercise for Dredging *Ren* and *Du* Channels. Loosen the body naturally after doing this exercise.

3.26 Daoyin Exercise for Dredging Ren and Du Channels (Tong Ren Du Daoyin Gong)

Function: Promotes free circulation of Qi within the Ren and Du channels and promotes proper circulation within all other channels.

Methods

1. **Preparation.** Stand erect with feet close together, with hands hanging naturally at the sides and the chin tucked in as if supporting an object on the head. Keep your eyes looking straight ahead, breathe evenly, and focus your mind on the *Dantian*. Stand this way for a short while.

2. **Activating the Coccyx (Weiluguan).** Bend forward at waist to form an angle of about 100 to 150. Interlock the fingers, rotate the palms outward (Fig. 55). Look straight ahead, but do not see anything. Breathe naturally and mentally to induce the movement of Qi from the *Dantian* to the coccyx. Swing the waist left and right from this position 36 times.

3. **Opening *Jiajiguan*.** Continuing from the last movement, bring yourself back to an upright position. Make a fist with the left hand and reach it out while the left foot stretches forward half a step. At the same time, pull the right arm back with the thumb pulled back and the other fingers forwards to form a posture like a warrior pulling a bow (Fig 56). Direct Qi mentally from the coccyx to the two *Jiajiguan* points, and swing the body left and right 36 times. Exchange hands and feet to swing for another 36 times.

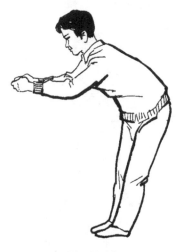

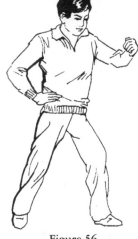

Figure 55   Figure 56

4. **Dredging Yuzhenguan.** Stand with feet shoulder-width apart. Interlace the fingers, raise the hands overhead, and cross the fingers with palms upwards (Fig. 57). Alternate the heels up and down 81 times, as if peddling something, and direct Qi to move from the coccyx *(Weiluguan)*, up the back, to *Jiajiguan*, *Yuzhenguan*, and finally to the Upper Dantien or Mud Ball.

5. **Returning to the *Diantian*.** From the last movement, cup one hand in the other in front of the chest and at the level of the point *Tanzhong* (Ren 17). Bend the knees to form a sitting posture (Fig 58). The height of this posture depends on the constitution of the individual performing the exercise. Direct Qi from the Upper *Dantian* along the *Ren* Channel down to the Lower *Dantian* and concentrate the mind on the Lower *Dantian*. Stand erect, allow the to fall naturally at the sides of the body. Finish the exercise by gently rubbing the hands and face and moving freely.

Application

With its function of regulating the *Ren* and *Du* Channels, this exercise is used mainly for health promotion. It may also be used as an auxiliary therapy to aid in the recovery of certain chronic diseases. In combination with Circulation Exercise and Inner Health Cultivation Exercise, this exercise is useful for developing and circulating Qi through the *Ren* and *Du* Channels. When Qi is circulating smoothly during Qigong practice, it can help clear up the *Ren* and *Du* Channels and prevent Qigong deviation.

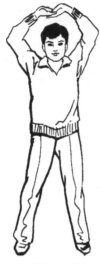

Figure 57

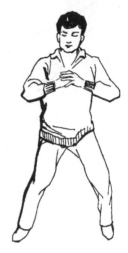

Figure 58

Points for Attention

Defecate before practice. The optimal time for practice is in the morning or at night after dynamic or static Qigong is performed. If you cannot feel Qi activity, maintain only mental activities. Long term practice will result in the ability to feel the movements of Qi.

CHAPTER 4

Emitting Outgoing Qi (Wai Qi)

4.1 Training of Qi

Training Qi is the first step in developing the ability to emit Qi. A Qigong doctor usually has to undergo long-term physical (dynamic) and internal (static) exercises before his Qi can be voluntarily regulated, replenished, and circulated down to the *Diantian*, and then circulated throughout the body and its channels. Wherever a Qigong doctor's mind is concentrated, there is Qi, and wherever there is Qi, there is strength. This is the foundation from which Qigong doctors emit outgoing Qi. Training Qi is mainly achieved through static exercises, dynamic exercises, and *Daoyin* self-massage.

4.1.1 STATIC EXERCISE FOR TRAINING QI.

Posture. A sitting, standing, or lying posture may be selected for the training of Qi. One may select the posture that is most suitable as the main posture and take the other ones as supplementary postures so that any opportunity for practice can be taken. The essentials and methods of posture training have been described in Chapter 2.

Respiration. Reverse abdominal respiration is the breathing strategy best suited for this training. Beginners may first practice natural respiration and then progress to abdominal respiration. When one is comfortable with breathing basics, they can shift to reverse respiration. The purpose of this respiration training is to make the breath become deep, long, fine, and even. This skill comes from a gradual accumulation of experience in respiration regulation. One cannot expect to master it overnight.

Mind Regulation. Setting the mind on the *Diantian* is the main method of mental concentration when training in static Qigong. The method is literally called concentration on point, which is practiced to open the small circulation *(Xiao Zhou Tian)* or the large circulation *(Da Zhou Tian)*.

Static Exercise Training Methods

Assume a proper posture, relax, and clear the mind of distractions. Imagine that the turbid Qi within the body is expelled through the mouth, nose, and pores during exhalation. During inhalation, imagine bringing fresh Qi into every aspect of the body. After three exhalations, tap the upper and lower teeth together 36 times then move the tongue within the mouth and swallow the accumulated saliva in three segments. Imagine that the clear Qi of heaven and earth joins the saliva as it descends to the *Dantian* and nourishes the whole body.

Smooth, even respiration along with concentration of the mind on the *Dantian* should be carried out in a natural and lively fashion. Voluntary holding of respiration and rigid mind concentration should be avoided.

Training of Qi should be combined with nourishing of Qi in every session. Conditions permitting, it is best to practice between 11:00 P.M. to 1:00 A.M and from 11:00 A.M. to 1:00 P.M. During the rest of the day, you can mainly practice nourishing of Qi. Training Qi requires focused attention and exercising by means of voluntary respiration and mind activities. Nourishing Qi refers to the experience of a static inner health cultivation state in which there is involuntary breathing and mind activities; respiration that is soothing, relaxed, natural and soft; and highly focused attention. During exercise, when you have entered quiescence by practicing reverse abdominal respiration and mind concentration on the Lower *Dantian* and when you have achieved a relaxed body breathing that is soft, even, and fine, you can start to do inner health cultivation. Only by combining training with nourishing can you achieve satisfactory results. This step can be called Qi Generating in the *Dantian* and Circulating All Over. After a certain period of practice, there will be noticeable Qi in the *Dantian* during exercise, and you may have a feeling of substantialness, warmth, movement of Qi, or other interesting but comfortable feelings. This sensation of Qi will become stronger and stronger as time goes by. When you have entered quiescence, the *Dantian* may feel hot, and you may experience a stream of warm air (Qi) rushing from the *Dantian* to the coccyx area. This rush of air will make you relaxed and comfortable all over. Sometimes the point *Huiyin* (Ren 1) will throb. When this happens, you should guide genuine Qi to circulate along the *Du* Channel towards the two pairs of Qigong gates *Jiajiguan* and *Yuzhenguan* and further, through *Baihui* (Du 20) and then along the *Ren* Channel down back to the coccyx. The principle of focusing attention merely when Qi has not started to move and leading it to circulate when it is about to move should be adhered to. To guide genuine Qi to flow in the *Ren* and *Du* Channels, mind concentration should be carried out in cooperation with breathing. When inhaling, conduct flow along the *Du* Channel; when exhaling, conduct it to flow along the *Ren* Channel back to the *Dantian*. This is traditionally called small circulation *(Xiao Zhou Tian)*. When you reach the quiescent state, gathered Qi will not disperse; it will circulate naturally along the *Ren* and *Du* Channels under the guidance of the mind without the help of breathing.

Carry out the closing process seriously after each exercising session. To perform the closing correctly, shift your mind slowly off the point you have been concentrating on, lead Qi to the Lower *Dantian*, relax yourself all over, open your eyes slowly, and do some self-massage.

Self-massage includes rubbing the hands, bathing the face (rubbing with palms), combing the hair with the fingertips, and dredging the 12 channels. Rubbing from the chest to the internal aspect of the hands, and along the medial aspect of the arm, will dredge the Three *Yin* Channels of the Hand. To dredge The *Yang* Channels of the Hand, rub from the outer aspect of the hands up to the shoulders and the lateral sides of the head and down the lateral aspect of the chest and abdomen. Rubbing from the waist and hips to the feet will dredge the Three *Yang* Channels of the Foot, and rubbing from the feet to the medial aspect of the abdomen will dredge the Three *Yin* Channels of the Foot. Repeat the above sequence 10 times. Limber yourself up to end the exercise.

4.1.2 DYNAMIC EXERCISE FOR TRAINING QI.

Dynamic exercise for training Qi lays the foundation for the ability to emit Qi. While static exercise gathers and strengthens Qi internally, dynamic exercise lays the foundation for guiding Qi by regulating the channels and strengthening the bones and muscles externally, thereby ensuring Qi to circulate freely.

Dynamic Exercise Training Methods

1. **Basic Posture.** Stand relaxed and quiet, with feet shoulder-width apart and toes clutching at the ground. Allow the hands to fall naturally at the sides. The head should be held as if it is supporting an object. Look straight ahead but see nothing, and place the tongue against the palate. Drop the shoulders and elbows. The chest should protrude slightly; pull the buttocks in slightly, and keep the knees relaxed and somewhat bent. Focus your mind and breathe naturally. After adjusting the posture, expel the turbid Qi three times by way of exhalation as done in static Qigong practice. Then bend and stretch the knees alternately to cause the legs and, perhaps even the whole body, to quiver and vibrate. The amplitude of vibration may

feel unnatural at first. After some practice, it will feel more natural, and the vibration will converge toward the *Dantian*. Eventually, the Qi will become the center of the vibration and the extremities will vibrate only slightly. This is called a pile driving vibration (natural with small amplitude). It is required for all the exercise forms described hereafter.

2. **Massaging the *Dai* Channel (The Belt Channel).** Proceed from the last stance. Place the palms on the right side of the *Dai* Channel, and massage it in cooperation with reverse abdominal respiration. During inhalation, push the Qi of the *Dai* Channel with the palms (the right is preceded by the left) to flow to the left. The mind should follow the palms. In order to try and sense internal activity, close the eyes slightly to achieve inward vision of the *Dai* Channel. During exhalation, push the Qi of the *Dai* Channel to flow to the right with the palms (the left is preceded by the right). All the other actions remain the same as above. Repeat this sequence for 9 respiratory cycles (Fig. 59). Carry out the same technique as above except this time during inhalation push the Qi of the *Dai* Channel to the right and during exhalation push the Qi of the *Dai* Channel to the left. Repeat this for another 9 respiratory cycles. Breathing, posture, and mind concentration should be well coordinated during practice. The waist should be relaxed to the utmost and should rotate in small amplitude along with the motion induced by hand manipulations. You may feel your waist as soft as silk, the *Dai* Channel warm, and the Qi flowing about the waist and circulating freely and vigorously all over the body.

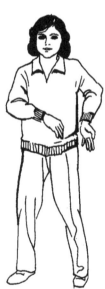

Figure 59

3. **Opening and Closing of the Three *Dantians*.** Assume the standing posture as explained in method one. When inhaling, extend the arms (elbows slightly bent) in front of the Lower *Dantian* with the backs of the palms facing each other (the point Outer *Laogong* (P 8) of each hand pointing at each other). Then slowly move the hands apart until they are shoulders-width apart. During this motion contract the abdomen and the anus. During exhalation, bring the hands back together so that

the Inner *Laogong* (P 8) of the hands faces the Lower *Dantian* and is the distance of one fist from it (Fig. 60). Perform the movement for 9 respiratory circles. Next, move the hands up to the level of the Middle *Dantian* (*Tanzhong* (Ren 17)) and perform this movement for 9 respiratory cycles. During inhalation lift the Qi to the Middle *Dantian*, and send the genuine Qi down to the Lower *Dantian* during exhalation. The last step is to open and close the Upper *Dantian*. Move the hands up to the Upper *Dantian* (the point *Yintang* (Extra 1)) and do the same hand movements as above for another 9 respiratory cycles. During the initial stages of practice, lift the hands to the Middle *Dantian* during inhalation and guide the Qi back to the Lower *Dantian* during exhalation. Qi can be conducted to the Upper *Dantian* gradually as the practice is carried on for a longer period of time.

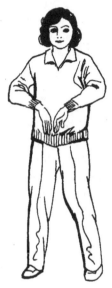

Figure 60

Important Points

The training of posture in the above exercises uses the standing vibrating posture as its basis. One must combine this posture with changes of posture to get Qi to move naturally with the movements of the exercise.

4.1.2.1 Double-Nine Yang Exercise

This exercise is similar to the famous Sinew Transforming Exercise. Certain posturing, proper breathing, and mind concentration are used to get Qi to circulate throughout the body. This exercise builds up the physique and activates its vitality. It is a fundamental skill for emitting Qi.

Beginning Double-Nine Yang Exercise

Form One: The Immortals Pointing Out the Way. Stand with your feet shoulder-width apart. Inhale, contract the abdomen and anus, and lift Qi from the Lower *Dantian* to the Middle *Dantian*. Simultaneously, move both hands upward to the sides of the waist with palms facing up and elbows bent. As you exhale, guide Qi to the right hand. The position of the right hand should be such that the four fingers of the hand are close together and the thumb stretched, the center of the palm hollowed and the joint of the wrist bent up a little.

When guiding Qi, direct internal strength to the arm, push the hand (palm erect) forward, and gather strength in the thenar eminence minor of the hand. As you inhale again, make a fist and draw it back to the chest. Open fist and face palm downward and press. Turn the left palm up and lift it to hold Qi up to the Middle *Dantian*. When exhaling, push the left hand forward in the same method as described for the right hand. Repeat the process 9 times for each hand. Finally return the hands to the front of the chest, and hold up to the Middle *Dantian*. Turn the palms to face each other in preparation for the next step (Fig. 61). Note: This form is used to train Qi of the *Shaoyin* and *Shaoyang* Channels. During exhalation, direct internal strength to the arm and push the hand out with the palm dented a little to gather strength in it. As you practice direct internal strength to the arm, palm, thenar eminence minor, and further to the small finger to make Qi pass all through the Channels of Hand *Shaoyin*

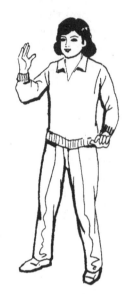

Figure 61

and Hand *Shaoyang*. Along with the vibrating, Qi will be continuously sent from the Lower *Dantian* and drawn back into it.

Form Two: Pushing Eight Horses Forward Proceed from the last stance. Exhale and direct Qi to the shoulders and arms. With the two palms facing each other, the thumbs stretched, and the four fingers of each hand close to each other, push the hands out slowly until the palms are at shoulder level. Bend the thumbs upward and pull them back. Depress the palms to make Qi fill the tips of the four fingers of each hand (Fig. 62). As you inhale, relax the extremities. Bend the thumbs upward and pull them back, bend the elbows slowly, and draw the hands back at the hypochondria. Repeat for 9 respiratory cycles. To end this sequence, draw the palms back and cross them in

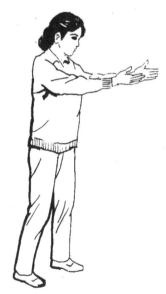

Figure 62

front of the chest. Note: This form is used to train the energy of the fingertips. Qi is directed mainly through the *Yangming* Channel of Hand *Taiyin* to the palms and the fingertips. A distending or hot sensation in the fingertips means that Qi has reached its destination.

Form Three: The Phoenix Spreading Its Wings Proceed from the last stance. Exhale and set the crossed palms apart from each other. Direct Qi to the two arms. Bend the fingers back (the four fingers close together) as if the Inner *Laogong* (P 8) was going to protrude. Face the back of the palms toward each other and push them apart until the hands, elbows, and the shoulders are at the same level. Fingers should remain still bent backward with the Inner *Laogong* (P 8) protruding (Fig. 63). Inhale. Turn the palms so that they face each other. Bend the elbows and slowly draw the palms together until they are again crossed in front of the chest. Draw them back to the sides of the chest to get prepared for the next step. Repeat for 9 respiratory cycles. Note: This form is aimed at training of the Channels of Hand *Jueyin* and Hand *Shaoyang*. Qi is accumulated in the Inner *Laogong* (P 8) when the hands are pushed out and in Outer *Laogong* (P 8) when the hands are pulled back and sent back to *Dantian*. As a result of persistent training of this form, the line of Qi will always be kept in the palms between the Inner and Outer *Laogong* (P 8). It is a very important form for guiding and emitting outgoing Qi.

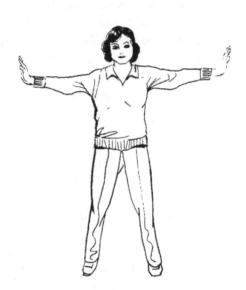

Figure 63

Form Four: Holding the Sky with the Hands Proceed from the last stance. Exhale while lifting the palms slowly. When they get to the point *Lianquan* (Ren 23), turn them outward slowly as you continue to lift them until they are above the head, as if holding something. The arms should be stretched and the fingertips of the two hands should point at each other about a fist apart. The fingers should be closed together with the thumbs abducted (Fig. 64). Inhale and rotate the wrists to get the fingertips pointing upward. Lower the hands until their

Inner *Laogong* (P 8) face the *Ren* Channel. Repeat for 9 respiratory cycles. To end this segment, place the hands at the sides of the chest with palms facing upward in preparation for the next step. Because the movements are long in both directions, you may inhale and exhale as necessary to keep yourself comfortable. Just be sure you are in full exhalation at the top of the movement and full inhalation at the end. Note: This form is aimed at training the Three *Yin* Channels of Hand. It can make Qi flow along the Three *Yin* Channels of Hand to the face of the palms, then along the Three *Yang* Channels of Hand downward.

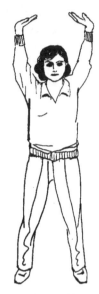

Figure 64

Form Five: Scooping the Moon from Water. Proceed from the last stance. Exhale and move the hands away from the sides of the body. Bend the body forward with the arms hanging loosely. Draw the hands between the feet with fingertips pointing at each other until they are one fist apart (Fig. 65). Accumulate energy at the fingertips as if holding a bulky weight. Inhale, straighten the waist naturally to hold the moon up to the sides of the chest, and direct Qi to the *Dantian*. Repeat the above process for 9 respiratory cycles. To end this segment, point the palms upward at the sides of the chest and prepare for the next step. Note: When bending forward, you should move your waist smoothly and slowly. The eyes should be closed slightly to look at the moon (a round object or a light mass or a tiny glittering spot that can be taken as the moon). The hands probe as if, trying to catch the moon and then holding it up to the *Dantian*. This exercise is good for nourishing genuine Qi, reinforcing the kidneys, and regulating both the *Ren* and the *Du* Channels.

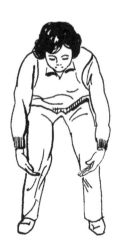

Figure 65

Form Six: Holding the Ball and Stroking It Three Times. Proceed from the last stance. Exhale while moving the hands to the right side of the body. Palms should be facing each other with the right hand above the left and as if holding a ball. While inhaling, pull the palms a little farther away from each other as if the ball were being inflated. Next, exhale and press the ball as if to compress the air inside it (Fig.66). Repeat the above for 3 respiratory cycles.

Rotating the palms simultaneously, bring the left hand above the right as if to turn the ball upside down in front of the abdomen. Repeat the inflating and compressing sequence for 3 respiratory cycles. Finally, shift hands to the left side of the body, and turn the ball upside down to get the right hand above the left. Repeat the inflating and compressing sequence for 3 respiratory cycles. Let hands stay at the left side for the next step. Note: This form is practiced to direct Qi to the palms to fill the six channels in the hand.

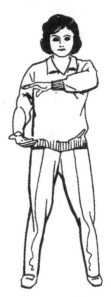

Figure 66

Form Seven: Moving the Palms As If Setting Tiles on the Roof. Proceed from the last posture. Inhale, stretch the left palm forward, and draw the right palm back. Then exhale and stretch the right palm forward, drawing the left palm back. (Fig. 67) Perform this sequence for 9 respiratory cycles. When the sequence is complete, move the hands to the sides of the chest with the palms facing up to prepare for the next segment. Note: This form is aimed at dredging the Three *Yin* and Three *Yang* Channels of the Hand to get Qi to reach the palms.

Form Eight: The Wind Swaying the Lotus Leaf. Proceed from the last stance. Exhale and stretch out the palms slowly until the palms and elbows are at shoulder level (Fig.68). Cross the palms with the left above the right and both palms facing upward. Inhale and slightly depress the thenar eminence to facilitate flow through the Hand *Taiyin* Channel to the tips of the thumbs. When exhaling, push out the thenar eminence

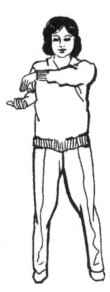

Figure 67

67

minor to facilitate flow along the Hand *Taiyang* Channel to the thenar and the tip of the little finger. When inhaling again, draw the hands back to the chest as in the starting position. Repeat this exercise for 9 or 18 respiratory cycles. To complete this segment bring the hands (palms upward) to the chest in preparation for the next form. Note: This form activates the channels of the Hand *Taiyin*, Hand *Taiyang*, Hand *Shaoyin*, and Hand *Shaoyang*, making the Qi of these Channels circulate continuously.

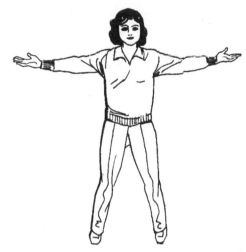

Figure 68

Form Nine: Regulating Qi All Over. Proceed from the last stance. Exhale and turn the palms so the fingertips point forward. Stretch the palms out until the shoulders, elbows, and wrists are at the same level (Fig. 69). Inhale and turn the hands so the backs of the palms are facing each other. Separate the palms to draw an arc with them, and lift Qi to the armpits (Fig. 70). The palms should be facing up and the fingertips of both hands point-ing to the sides of the chest. Stretch the palms out again when exhaling, ready to draw another arc. Repeat this sequence for 9 or 18 respiratory cycles. Note: This form combines heaven, earth, and human into an organic whole and regulates the Qi of the whole body in preparation for the final form.

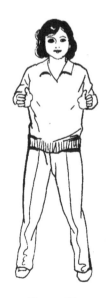
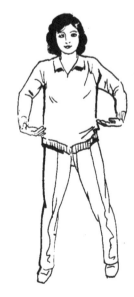

Figure 69   Figure 70

Closing Form of Double-Nine *Yang* Exercise. Overlap the two hands (right over the left for men, vice versa in females). Apply them to the lower *Dantian*. Stop vibrating gradually and restore equilibrium. Breathe naturally and concentrate on the *Dantian* for a while. Rub your hands and face and move freely to end the exercise.

4.1.2.2 Exercise of Kneading the Abdomen to Strengthen the Active Substance in the Body.

This exercise is an auxiliary to static and dynamic Qigong for training Qi. Practicing it in combination with static and dynamic exercises can strengthen internal organs, and reinforce intrinsic Qi. This exercise also serves to increase strength and can avoid any risk of deviations due to undesirable opening and closing of the points. This is especially important to those who are versed in Qigong practice and who carry out treatment of patients by emitting outgoing Qi. If they treat patients and do not practice these kinds of exercises, they may become insufficient in active substance, deficient in Qi, and weak in strength. If they emit outgoing Qi to treat patients, their health will be easily impaired by pathogens because they are not strong enough internally to prevent their points from improper opening resulting in lowered resistance to external pathogenic factors. This can cause local discomfort or a morbid physical state, which can lead to a general disorder of activities, and eventual collapse of the achievements gained through long-term practice. Kneading the Abdomen to Strengthen the Active Substance is not only an auxiliary exercise for strengthening the intrinsic Qi, but indispensable for those who treat patients with outgoing Qi.

Methods

Lie supine on the bed with both legs stretched naturally and hands at the sides of the body. The whole body (especially the viscera) should be relaxed. Dispel distracting thoughts, and breathe naturally with the tongue pressed against the palate.

Place one palm (the right palm for males and the left palm for females) on the abdomen under the xiphoid process and rotate the palm clockwise for males and counterclockwise for females to knead the upper abdomen. Do not exert force intentionally or let the hand get stiff. The correct manipulation should be natural and gentle and should give a soft sensation under the palm inside the upper abdomen. Avoid distractions, keep inward vision attentively, and concentrate the mind on the Middle *Dantian*. One should neither forget the flow of Qi or speed up its flow; simply let it progress naturally. Maintain natural breath with a calm mind, and try to get the pleasant feeling of warm, gentle, and continuously flowing Qi under the palm. Each practice session should last 15–30 minutes. The time can be increased gradually to one hour but over-fatigue of the arm should be avoided. Carry out the kneading three times a day—in the morning, at noon, and in the evening—or twice a day—in the morning and evening.

After practicing about a month, as Qi accumulates gradually, you may feel that your stomach is consolidated and your appetite and sleep improved. You may also have the feeling of Qi in the mid-upper abdomen when it is pressed. The straight muscles of the abdomen may gradually become more solid or bulged, which may appear more clearly when you direct or exert strength to it. In this stage, the midline from the xiphoid process to the navel may be still soft and dented indicating that in the *Ren* Channel is still not substantial. To improve it, massage the midline with your palm and strike along it gently with a hollow fist. The dent will eventually disappear, as the Qi in the *Ren* Channel will become more substantial. This goal usually takes a hundred days to attain.

As a following step, perform clockwise kneading to the right side of the abdomen in a spiral fashion from under the ribs down to the groin. Use the right palm first. Repeat 12 times. Do the same movement, 12 times counterclockwise, with the left palm on the left abdomen. When this is complete, with the right palm, massage the lower abdomen where the Lower *Dantian* is located in a circular manner for 15–30 minutes. Next, pat the same area with a hollow fist for a comfortable period of time. By doing so, the Qi, and the whole abdomen, will become substantial and will be strong and solid in about a hundred days. When you have completed massaging the abdomen, the next step is to strike on the midline and right and left sides of the chest with a hollowed fist in the manner described above. Long-term practice of this exercise will make both the chest and the abdomen substantial, indicating that both the *Ren* and *Chong* Channels are full of Qi.

At this stage, you can direct Qi into the *Du* Channel and ask someone to pat along it, and along the first and second collaterals of the Urinary Bladder Channel, up and down and vice versa. Then ask the assistant to rub these places with his or her palm in order to get Qi even and full. In this way, the *Du* Channel will be substantial with in about a hundred days.

When the *Ren* and *Du* Channels are filled with consolidated Qi, you can carry out patting yourself on the upper and lower extremities from top to bottom, with emphasis on the regions where there are plumpy muscles. The patting or striking of other parts can be done with the palm, a hollow fist or a specially made wooden hammer. With about one year's practice of Kneading the Abdomen to Strengthen the Active Substance in the Body, you may feel that you are full of substantial Qi and vigorous all over. Your resistance to external pathogenic factors will be strong, your points will be opened and closed desirably and will not be affected by turbid Qi. From that point on, you can take some time every day to do the kneading of the abdomen and patting on the extremities to maintain proper circulation and substance.

4.2 The Guiding of Qi

Guiding or directing Qi means to guide intrinsic Qi to a certain part of the body where outgoing Qi is emitted. This ability is usually possible only when one has undergone serious, long-term training. When guiding Qi, one should have the Qi follow the mind and should be able to control and feel the direction, pattern, nature, and amount of intrinsic Qi. The following exercise is aimed at laying solid foundations for emitting Qi through the hands.

4.2.1 STANDING VIBRATING WITH PALMS CLOSED TO GUIDE QI.

1. **Posture.** Assume the standing, pile-driving, vibrating posture. Keep the feet shoulder-width apart, and bend the arms to place the palms together in front of the chest. The fingertips should be pointing upward and elbows and wrists at the same level. Imagine yourself supporting an object on the head. Tuck in the chest, and straighten the back, and relax the hips and knees. Rest the tongue on the palate, and close the eyes slightly (Fig 71).

2. **Guiding.** Breathe naturally and concentrate on the *Dantian*. When you feel the movement of internal energy (a sensation of warmth and circulation), exhale and have your mind follow it into the *Du* Channel, through the Three *Yang* Channels of the Hand, and into the palms and fingertips. When inhaling, guide the Qi back to the *Dantian* along the same channels. When Qi is circulating freely, keep your atten-

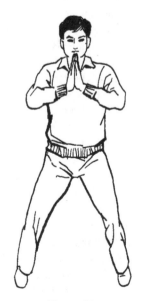

Figure 71

71

tion on the palms and the fingertips with gentle natural breathing. Your palms will feel hot and your fingertips will feel thicker and distended. A tingling sensation and slight vibration, as if something were coming out of the hands, will also occur. Practice this exercise once or twice a day, 5–10 minutes each time.

4.2.2 SINGLE FINGER MEDITATION TO GUIDE QI.

1. **Posture.** Assume the standing, pile-driving, vibrating posture. The left hand should be lifted to the left shoulder level. Keep the wrist bent, the index finger straight and the rest of the fingers curved. The tips of the thumb and the middle finger should touch each other to form a ring. The right hand (in the same gesture as the left) is at the right side of the abdomen and the index fingers of the two hands point at each other (Fig. 72).

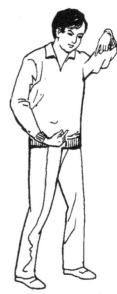

2. **Guiding.** Breathe naturally and concentrate the attention on the *Dantian*. As soon as the Qi in the *Dantian* is activated, begin to breathe slowly and direct the Qi to the tip of the right index finger. When you feel energy has reached this point (you will feel your fingertip hot and distending as if something is being released from it), then direct the Qi to the tip of the index finger of the left hand. When you feel that there is attractive force between the tips of the two fingers, begin to rap with the tip of the left index finger on the energetic column being emitted from the right. You will get a strong feeling of Qi in the two hands. Next,

Figure 72

direct Qi to the left index finger to emit it toward the right hand and repeat the rapping movement. Switch hand positions so the right hand is over the left and repeat the above. Practice this exercise once or twice a day, 5–30 minutes each time.

4.2.3 PALM-PUSHING AND PALM-PULLING TO GUIDE QI.

1. **Posture.** Assume the standing, pile-driving, vibrating posture. Allow the fingers of both hands to separate naturally. Stretch the right hand naturally forward to the right and bend the left arm so that the left hand is in front of the chest. The center of the

two palms should face each other (Fig. 73). Assume the same posture when the position of the two hands is exchanged.

2. **Guiding.** Breathe naturally and concentrate the mind on the *Dantian*. When the Qi in the *Dantian* is activated, push the palms toward each other, leading the Qi to the Inner *Laogong* (P 8) of the left palm and emitting it towards the Inner *Laogong* (P 8) of the right palm. Stop pushing to accumulate Qi between the palms, and draw the palms back to the original position. As the palms move apart, you should feel as if you are stretching Qi. You will get strong feeling of Qi when doing this part of the sequence. Exchange hands and repeat the procedure. This exercise may be practiced once or twice a day, 5–30 minutes each time.

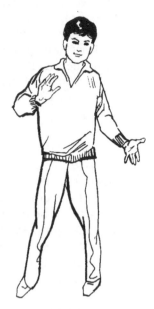

Figure 73

4.2.4 MAKING THREE POINTS LINEAR TO GUIDE QI.

1. **Posture.** Light an incense stick, and put the incense burner on the table. You can also use a similar object such as a flower or a tree as the point of focus. Assume the standing, pile-driving, vibrating posture. Stretch the right palm naturally in front of the incense with the burning tip of the incense pointing at inner *Laogong* (P 8) of the palm. The left hand should assume the Single Finger-meditation gesture (exercise 4.2.2). Place the finger behind the tip of the burning incense with the fingertip pointing at the incense tip. The three points—the left index fingertip, the tip of the burning incense and the Inner *Laogong* (P 8) of the right palm— should form a line (Fig. 74).

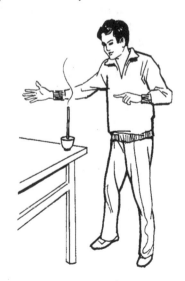

2. **Guiding.** Proceed from the last stance. Breathe naturally and concentrate the attention on the *Diantian*. When the Qi in the

Figure 74

Dantian is activated, direct the energy to the tip of the left index finger. Exhale lightly, slowly, and fully and focus attention on the incense tip. Continue to emit Qi and send it further toward the right hand. You will have strong feeling of Qi in the Inner *Laogong* (P 8) of the right hand. During each inhalation allow the Qi accumulate in the *Dantian*. This exercise may be practiced once or twice a day, 5–30 minutes each time.

4.2.5 MAKING THREE POINTS CIRCULAR TO GUIDE QI

1. **Posture.** Assume the standing, pile-driving vibrating posture. Light an incense stick and place it in a holder on a table. As in the last exercise, you can take a similar object such as a flower or a tree as the focus point. Open the two hands naturally to form an equilateral triangle using three points—the two points Inner *Laogong* (P 8) of both palms and the tip of the burning incense. Mentally draw a circle surrounding the triangle (Fig. 75). Qi will fill the circle as you progress in your practice.

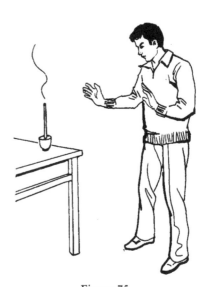

Figure 75

2. **Guiding.** Allow your breathing to remain natural, and concentrate your attention on the *Dantian*. When Qi in the *Dantian* is activated, lead it to the Inner *Laogong* (P 8) of both hands. Exhale lightly, slowly, and deeply to emit Qi towards the incense tip. Make the three points attract or support one another. Imagine yourself holding a ball with your hands. Move your hands in response to the sensation of Qi. While one hand pulls, the other pushes or vice versa. This exercise may be practiced once or twice a day, 5–30 minutes each time.

4.2.6 JUMPING TO GUIDE QI IN BURSTS.

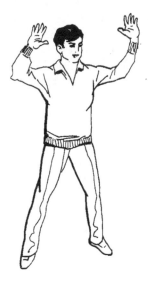

Figure 76

1. Posture. Stand with feet shoulders-width apart, bend the knees slowly, and make fists to gather Qi. Inhale and concentrate your attention on the *Dantian*. When exhaling, jump straight up and stretch the hands out in front of the chest with the fingers separated and the palms facing forward as if they were spreading claws (Fig. 76).

2. Guiding. During inhalation, concentrate your attention on the Qi in the *Dantian*. Lift Qi to the chest and gather it in the palms. When exhaling (as you jump), concentrate your attention on the center of the palms allowing the Qi to burst out from the Inner *Laogong* (P 8). This exercise may be practiced once or twice a day, 24 or 48 respiratory cycles each time.

4.2.7 GUIDING QI IN FIXED FORM.

1. Posture. Sit on or stand by a bed. Rest the left hand naturally on the left knee and put the right hand on the bed. The periphery of the palm should touch the bed but suspend the center of the palm above it. Allow the shoulders and elbows to drop, and keep the elbows slightly bent. The wrists should remain relaxed.

2. Guiding Qi. Breathe evenly and concentrate your attention on the *Dantian*. When the Qi in the *Dantian* is activated, move the waist gently counterclockwise or clockwise. When inhaling, lift Qi to the chest. The intrinsic Qi should vibrate and move upward, little by little, and finally reach the palms. When exhaling, the vibration of the intrinsic Qi should vibrate the palms rhythmically. The frequency and force of the vibration will change with the level of mind concentration. When Qi reaches the palm, it will fill the palm and you will feel as if there is an ball inflating under your hand. The Qi should always be centered on the Inner *Laogong* (P 8) gathering together without dispersion. You should guide the energy generated in this exercise through the different hand forms associated with emitting Qi. The motion of Qi and the movements of the hand should always be in perfect harmony.[Refer to section 4.3.1 for information about the hand positions required for the training of guiding in vibration fixed form They include Middle Finger Propping *(Zhong Zhi Du Li Shi)* Spreading Claw *(Tan Zhua Shi)*, Sword-Thrust *(Jian Jue Shi)* and Dragon Mouth *(Long Xian Shi)*]. When you can feel the vibration in the right hand, switch and try the left. After some practice, you will be able to train the Qi to circulate in different frequencies and intensities. This exercise may be practiced 1–2 times a day, 30–60 minutes each time. Generally, it takes 3 months to develop skill in this exercise.

4.2.8 GUIDING QI SPIRALLY.

1. Posture. Any of the three postures (standing, sitting, or lying) will suffice for this exercise. The standing posture, however, is used as an example throughout the following description. Stand with feet shoulders-width apart and place the right hand in front of the right side of the chest with the elbow bent, palm facing forward, and fingertips pointing upward. Allow the left hand to hang naturally at the side, rest on the knees (if sitting) or under the navel (if lying).

2. Guiding. Allow the Qi in the *Dantian* to turn spirally in a counterclockwise direction inside the body through the chest and the upper extremities to the palms (remember the Qi should follow the mind concentration). With the navel as the center point in the *Dantian* and the *Laogong* (P 8) the center in the palms, use the mind to make the spiral synchronous. Beginners should start slowly and increase the speed of the spiral gradually. The spinning size of the spiral is flexible; you can visualize it increasing or decreasing in size as it moves. This exercise requires patience. Do not be too anxious for quick results. The skill of guiding cannot be mastered overnight. You must do the exercise frequently, making full use of all three postures. Be sure to train both hands equally.

4.2.9 COLD AND HEAT GUIDANCE OF QI.

This guiding exercise conforms to the TCM principle of treating the cold syndrome with hot-natured drugs and the heat syndrome with cold-natured drugs. Heat guidance of Qi primarily requires proper posture adjustment, even breathing, and concentration of the mind on the *Dantian*. Imagine that the Qi in the *Dantian* is as hot as the burning sun shining all over the body. Shift this heat sensation to the palms as if the hot sun was burning there and giving off heat from the palms, fingertips, or through other hand gestures.

Cold guidance of Qi should also begin with proper posture adjustment, regulation of breathing, and concentration of mind on the *Dantian*. In this exercise, you should also concentrate on the point *Yongquan* (K 1). Inhale the earthly Qi by way of the heels, and direct it to the chest and palms. Imagine that the centers of the palms are as cold as ice and concentrate the mind on the coldness there. You should not imagine that your whole body is cold or direct the cold feeling to any other location lest it affect the coordination of activities. The exercise can be done together with other guiding exercises after you have mastered them.

Final Note. Of the above nine forms of exercises for guiding Qi, two or three can be selected for practice each time. After each session, you should stand calmly for a moment, direct Qi back to the *Dantian*, rub your hands and face, and move about freely for a while to end the exercise.

4.3 Emission of Qi

Emission of Qi is also called the emitting method *(Fa Gong)*, emitting of outgoing *Qi (Fafang Wai Qi)*, and in ancient times, distributing Qi *(Bu)*. It is a method practiced by those experienced in the training and guiding of Qi who can direct their intrinsic Qi to the palms, fingertips, or through other hand gestures and emit the Qi into the channels or points of another person.

4.3.1 HAND GESTURES FOR EMITTING QI.

1. Single Finger Meditation *(Yi Zhi Chan Shi)*. In this gesture, the index finger is stretched while the others are bent naturally. The thumb is bent gently over the back of the middle finger (Fig. 77). When using this gesture for emission, the Qi is guided to the tip of the index finger and is emitted through direct touch or by placing the index finger above the area being treated.

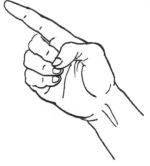

Figure 77

2. **Flat Palm** *(Ping Zhang Shi)*. Stretch the
   five fingers naturally (Fig 78). Direct Qi to
   the palm; the Inner *Laogong* (P 8) is the
   center through which the Qi will be emitted.
   The Qi is emitted through direct touch or by
   placing the palm above the area being
   treated.

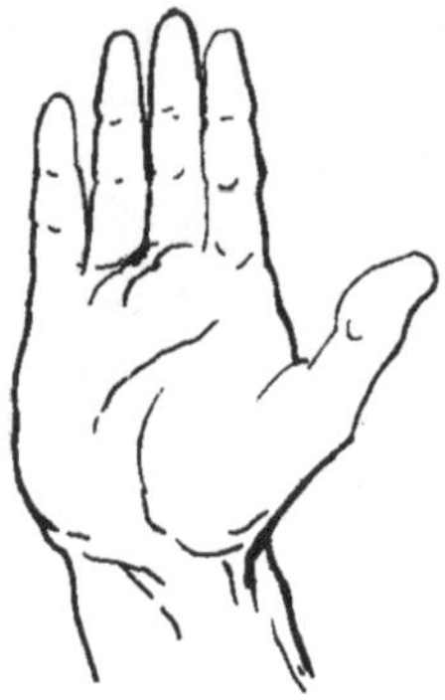

3. **Spreading Claw** *(Tan*
   Zhua Shi). Separate
   the fingers naturally
   and bend them as if
   grasping something
   (Fig. 79). Direct the
   Qi to the fingertips; it
   is emitted through
   direct contact or by
   placing the claw above
   the area being treated.

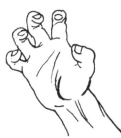

Figure 79

Figure 78

4. **Sword Thrust** *(Jian Jue Shi)*. With the
   index and middle fingers kept close together,
   allow the ring and small fingers to bend
   naturally. Place the thumb gently on nails of
   the bent fingers (Fig. 80). Direct the Qi to
   the tips of the index and middle fingers. The
   Qi is emitted through direct contact or by
   placing the fingers above the area being
   treated.

Figure 80

5. **Middle Finger Propping** *(Zhong Zhi Du Li*
   Shi). Stretch the middle finger and allow the
   rest of the fingers to bend naturally with the
   thumb touching the index finger (Fig 81).
   Direct Qi to the tip of the middle finger. The
   Qi is emitted through
   direct contact or by
   placing it above the area
   treated.

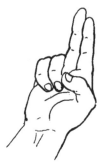

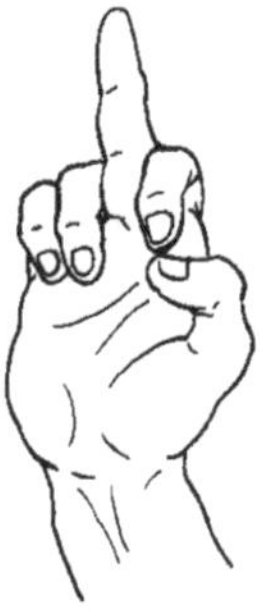

Figure 81

6. **Dragon Mouth** *(Long*
   Xian Shi). Keep the four
   fingers close to each other
   pointing straight and
   separated from the thumb
   (Fig. 82). Direct Qi to the
   locality between the thumb and the four fingers, and emit Qi
   towards the area being treated.

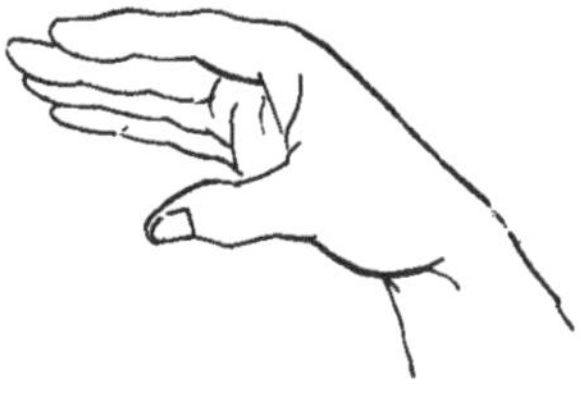

Figure 82

4.3.2 HAND MANIPULATIONS FOR EMITTING QI.

4.3.2.1 Manipulations with Hand Touching the Area Being Treated

Vibrating. Select a proper hand gesture. Lay the hand gently on the part to be treated and make vibrations (as explained in the previous section) to emit Qi. The vibrating method requires you to exert will to adjust the frequency, amplitude, nature, and amount of *Li* (power associated with muscular stimulation) and Qi emitted during session.

Kneading. Select a proper hand gesture or use the tip of the thumb to perform forceful rotary kneading. Kneading should be firm but should not cause discomfort on selected points or around the affected area. While kneading simultaneously guide and emit Qi.

Rubbing. Select a proper hand gesture or—with the four fingers close together—perform rotary massage slowly and forcefully on the selected points while guiding and emitting Qi.

Scrubbing. Using the flat palm or the flat of the four closed fingers, slowly scrub in a straight line the affected part while guiding and emitting Qi.

Pressing. Select a proper hand gesture. Place the hand on the affected part. Press vertically while guiding and emitting Qi.

4.3.2.2 Manipulations with Hand off the Area Being Treated.

Pushing. Select a proper hand gesture. Position the hand about 15–100 cm off the region being treated. Guide Qi as described in Making Two or Three Points Linear or Making Three Points Circular (sections 4.2.4 and 4.2.5). When you get the proper sensation, push your hand gently with internal strength so as to emit Qi to the affected region or related points.

Pulling. Select a proper hand gesture. Position the hand 15–100 cm off the region to be treated. Using the methods described in sections 4.2.4 and 4.2.5, guide Qi slowly to the affected area or related points. When you get Qi sensation, pull your hand gently with internal strength to emit Qi to the affected area.

Rotating. Select a proper hand gesture. Position the hand 15–100 cm off the region to be treated. Apply the Spiral Guiding method to arouse Qi slowly (section 4.2.8). When you feel Qi, conduct a spiral hand manipulation clockwise or counterclockwise so that it will flow in a spiral to the affected area or into the related points. You can also slowly guide Qi with the method described in sections 4.2.4 and 4.2.5. When you get the sensation of Qi, pull one hand and push the other gently and with internal strength making a circular motion to emit to the affected area.

Quivering. Select a proper hand gesture, and keep the hand 15–100 cm above the region being treated. Adopt the method Guiding Qi in Fixed Form (section 4.2.7) to guide Qi slowly. When you get the feeling of Qi, quiver the hand lightly to emit Qi to the region being treated or to the related points.

Leading. Select a proper hand posture, and place the hand 15–100 cm off the region being treated. When you feel the sensation of Qi, emit it toward the affected area and lead the energy to flow with or against the direction of the channels. You may also move to the left or right or up and down depending on the severity of the illness. Picking the right movement requires some understanding of TCM theory.

Locating. Select a proper hand posture and place the hand 15–100 cm off the region being treated. When you feel the sensation of Qi, use one or several emitting methods to make a fixed emission towards the area being treated.

4.3.2.3 Auxiliary Manipulations.

Tapping. Using one finger or the thumb, index, and middle fingers closed together, tap along the channels or on related acupuncture points.

Patting. With the empty palm (fingers naturally stretched), pat on the disordered region, along the channels, or on related points.

Hitting. Using a hollow fist, hit with its back or other parts on the disordered region, along the channels, or on related points.

Pressing in Intervals. Press with the tip of the thumb or the palm, in intervals, on the disordered region, along the channels, or on related points.

Stroking. Push and stroke with one or both palms along the channels, on related points, or on the affected region.

Plucking. Pluck the selected points with the fingers.

Rubbing Back and Forth. Press on the selected part from both sides using the two palms or with the flat of the thumbs and the index and middle fingers. Rub the part gently back and forth, exerting force symmetrically.

Rocking. Rock or pull (back and forth) the joints of the extremities.

Rolling. Using the back of the hand, roll on the region being treated. When performing rolling, the wrist joint should be bent, stretched, and turned repeatedly.

4.3.3 THE FORMS OF QI EMISSION.

Clinical experience in emitting Qi has indicated that, one of the keys to success in treatment with outgoing Qi is to use different forms to emit Qi according to the needs of the person being treated. There are three basic forms that are used when emitting Qi; they are: linear, fixed and spiral. Having grasped the three forms, one can apply them flexibly during clinical treatment in agreement with the conditions of the illness. You may apply one form, two forms in combination, or develop some special forms based on all three. The application of the three basic forms can be put into practice in combination with the hand gestures and manipulations, as well as with the method of cold and heat guidance to form a combined guiding, emitting process.

1. **Linear Form Emission.** The Two Point Line Method, Three Point Line Method (section 4.2.4) or other similar guiding methods are taken as the basic skills in training the linear form of emission. Pushing, pulling, locating, leading, and other hand manipulations are generally used to emit while using this form. The linear form of emission is mild and gives a clear sensation of constriction, tugging, and warmth or coldness. It is a basic form to induce channel Qi movement, supplement its deficiency, and purge its excess. This form requires the hand manipulation of emitting to be stable and slow and the breathing to be deep and natural.

2. **Fixed Form Emission.** This is a common emitting form, which uses the Vibrating and Fixed Guiding Method (sections 4.2.1 and 4.2.7) as the basic skills. It can be conducted using various hand manipulations. The fixed form gives marked stimulation to the Qi activities in the channels, points, and *Dantian*. It is a major form of mobilizing and stimulating Qi activity. This method usually requires one to take an upright sitting posture or a horse-riding stance while using natural and slow breathing. Using the waist as the axle and the abdomen as the pump, the inside of the body should vibrate as the Qi is guided to the part of the hand, which is emitting the Qi. The Qi should be emitted like pearls on a string. The mind should follow the vibration of the flow and give it guidance. When carrying out fixed emission of Qi, one must remember not to hold the breath or make the hand vibrate by vibrating the muscles. Otherwise, stagnation will occur and result in stuffiness in the chest, pain in the hypochondria, sharp pain in the arms (as if having a fracture), or laceration of the muscles. To have a good grasp of this emitting method, one should first master the vibrating method to ensure that Qi is emitted naturally. Generally, one should carry out the exercises in the following order: training, guiding, and vibrating Qi. Developing skill in this method of emitting is not an easy thing. One can expect to have a basic grasp of this form in

three months through diligent exercise. However, one cannot expect to apply it skillfully to clinical treatment without much longer practice.

3. **Spiral Form Emission.** This form utilizes the Guiding Qi Spirally method (section 4.2.8) as a way of emitting Qi. Qi moves spirally towards the affected area and penetrates deeply. It provides the special functions of regulating physiological activities. In this form, Qi is induced by natural respiration and spiral mind concentration. The Qi should start whirling from the vortex in the *Dantian* and move to the part of the hand from where it will be emitted. Learning this skill requires constant practice of rotation in the *Dantian* as well as the synchronization of the rotation with the hand gestures. It is essential to form a fixed spiral route of flowing Qi so that, when rotation begins in the *Dantian*, it will also whirl through the hand gesture. The flow of Qi should be regulated with the mind. Only after these abilities are attained, can one start applying this method to clinical treatments.

4.3.4 THE SENSATION OF QI.

The sensation of Qi refers to the response felt by both Qigong doctors and patients during Qigong treatment. A Qigong doctor can diagnose the patient's disease and adjust the procedures of treatment according to his feeling as well as the patient's feeling of Qi.

1. **The Sensation of Genuine Qi.** The sensation of genuine Qi is often manifested as a slightly warm, cold, tingling, constricting, flowing, or dragging sensation. In most cases, the direction, density, nature, and volume of the genuine Qi can be sensed.

2. **The Sensation of Filthy Qi.** The sensation of filthy is also referred to as the pathogenic message, which is different from the pathogenic factors of infectious disease found in modern medicine. Pathogenic message in Qigong terms can be classified as:

Cold Feeling. The Qi felt is especially cold. It may be so cold that when one gets such feeling, his fingertips get cold immediately, the terminal blood vessels will contract rapidly, and the coldness will transmit from the fingertips upwards, causing shivering and contraction of the pores.

Feeling of Dryness-Heat. This pathogenic message is felt on the body or hands of the Qigong doctor. The sensation may be a feeling of dryness-heat making him restless as if he were near a fire and being scorched.

Feeling of Soreness and Numbness. When such feeling occurs, one will experience local numbness and discomfort.

Filthy Qi can be felt when the Qigong doctor is standing or sitting opposite the patient or when the doctor is emitting towards the patient. It gives the Qigong doctor an unbearable offensive feeling. It is said that, since the ancient times, there have existed five kinds of internal pathogenic Qi such as joy and sorrow and six external pathogenic factors such as heat and wind. Sometimes a pathogenic factor can be sensed exactly if the Qigong doctor is quite attentive.

4.3.5 THE EFFECTS OF QI IN PATIENTS.

When Qigong doctors emits Qi to treat patients, most patients feel the following effects.

1. **Sensitive Effect.** When a Qigong doctor emits Qi, some patients may immediately or gradually get a feeling similar to that which occurs during Qigong practice such as cold, hot, depressing, towing, creeping, tingling, heavy, light, floating or sinking. This sensation represents a kind of effect occurring when Qi circulates in the channels and acts on affected areas to reach its focus. These feelings represent the sensitive effect.

2. **Dynamic Effect.** When a doctor emits Qi, the patient may immediately or gradually show involuntary movement of a certain part of the extremities or of the whole body. Some patients may have mild muscular tremor, others may get movements of the extremities in large amplitude. Such involuntary movements represent the dynamic effect.

3. **Photoelectric Effect.** When receiving outgoing Qi, some patients may feel a sensation of electric shock in the extremities. Others, with their eyes closed mildly, may see pictures of different shapes—most of which are circular, patchy, or lightning like. Such sensations are known as the photoelectric effect.

4. **Sound Effect.** Some patients may hear sounds such as "La-La," "Long-Long," or "Zhi-Zhi" when they receive outgoing Qi.

5. **Smell Effect.** Some patients may smell a special odor when receiving outgoing Qi and treatment. The odor varies in different patients. It may be the fragrance of sandalwood or that of flowers.

6. **Syncope Induced by Qiqong.** When receiving Qigong, a few patients may sweat all over and have faster heart rates than can be seen in fainting from acupuncture. Some patients may get syncope (fainting) although they may have no apparent sensation of Qi as a dynamic phenomenon. In some, illness may

improve markedly after they have experienced syncope. If syncope occurs, the Qigong doctor should make the patient lie supine and perform digital tapping on the points *Baihui* (Du 20), *Mingmen* (Du 4), *Jianjing* (G.B. 21), and *Yintang* (Extra 1), and do grasping manipulation on *Jianjing* (G.B. 21). The doctor should then conduct Qi along the *Ren* and *Du* Channels so it returns to its origin. The patient will then recover quickly.

Of the sensations mentioned above those described as Sensitive Effect occur most frequently. The Dynamic Effect occurs in a few patients, and the other phenomena occur very rarely. These responses to Qi represent a special state of the sense and motion organs in the patients who have received the outgoing Qi treatment. It is a factor that depends on the sensitivity of the sense organs and the channels of the patient rather than the pure therapeutic effect produced by working on the diseased site. Some patients may show no apparent effect but recover very quickly after several courses of treatment and gain sensation of Qi gradually. Some may have no marked improvement, yet they may experience a strong reaction. This is indeed a rather complicated problem, which awaits further studies.

4.3.6 THE CLOSING FORM OF QI EMISSION.

The Closing Form for Patients. When the Qigong doctor emits Qi to the patient, the patient may respond involuntarily as if he or she were also doing the exercises. When the treatment is over, the doctor should relax the patient by restoring the patient's Qi to its origin by means of hand manipulations (such as digital tapping, patting, percussing, rubbing, and rocking) as the conditions require.

The Closing Form for Qigong Doctors. To stop emitting, the Qigong doctor should direct his or her Qi slowly back to the *Dantian* and draw the hands off the emitting gesture. The doctor should then readjust the mind, breathing, and posture and bring genuine Qi back to its origin. If affected by pathogenic Qi, the doctor should first expel it and then carry out the readjustment.

CHAPTER 5

Treatment

5.1 Deviation of Qigong

Deviation of Qigong refers to the adverse reactions that can occur during the course of Qigong exercise. The practitioner may feel uncomfortable and may not be able to regain balance. Such reactions can be physically and mentally harmful. Common causes of deviation include:

- Exercising or practicing under the guidance of an inexperienced instructor or one who has no understanding of TCM theories
- Failing to obey the principle of exercising in light of concrete conditions such as those who are not fit for the exercise of intrinsic circulation but force themselves to do it anyway
- Hoping to experience quick results and thereby failing to respond to the effects of Qi in the correct way
- Failing to master the principle and methods of the Three Regulations leading to mental and physical confusion
- Becoming frightened or irritated during the course of Qigong practice
- Blindly or unnaturally guiding intrinsic Qi to circulate or force Qi to go out
- Becoming confused or suspicious concerning the normal phenomena occurring in the course of Qigong exercise
- Receiving treatment from an unqualified practitioner which can lead to deranged circulation of Qi

5.1.1 DERANGED FLOW OF QI.

Symptoms. Dizziness, vertigo, panic, chest distress, short breath, uncontrolled movement of the extremities, tremors of the body, continuous, uncomfortable flow of Qi along a particular channel or area.

Treatment

1. **Self-Treatment with Qigong Exercise.** Terminate the Qigong exercises that caused the symptoms mentioned above. Do not panic, and calm down the mind. Pat the areas where

the signs and symptoms are occurring and carry out self-massage along the proper route and in the correct direction. Massage the following channels: The Three *Yin* Channels of the Hand, The Three *Yin* Channels of the Foot, The Three *Yang* Channels of the Hand, and The Three *Yang* Channels of the Foot. If the symptoms are severe, see an experienced Qigong doctor.

2. **Treatment with Outgoing Qi.** Select points, in the locations and along the channels, where functional activities of have been in a state of disorder. Flat Palm or Sword Thrust hand gestures, as well as pushing, pulling and quivering manipulations, should be used to help normalize the functional activities of Qi along the disordered or related channels. To finish, use the pushing manipulation to regulate the *Yin* and *Yang* and to guide Qi to a certain channel, viscera, or *Dantian*.

5.1.2 STAGNATION OF QI AND STASIS OF BLOOD

Symptoms. Pain, heaviness, sore and distending sensation, and sensation of compression. These symptoms will not disappear automatically and may become worse if not treated.

1. **Self-Treatment with Qigong Exercise.** Terminate the Qigong exercises that have caused the symptoms.

If you feel a compressing sensation on the head and a severe headache, you may massage the acupuncture points *Baihui* (Du 20), *Fengfu* (GB 20), *Tianmen*, *Kangong*, and *Tajyang* (Extra 2) and then pat and massage along the route and direction of the *Du* and *Ren* Channels. When you have finished, concentrate the mind on *Yongquan* (K 1) and *Dadun*(Liv 1) and carry out Head and Face Exercise.

If you feel tight and compressed on the forehead, you may first massage the points *Tianmen*, *Kangong*, and *Taiyang* (Extra 2) and then pat from *Baihui* (Du 20) down to the *Dantian* along the *Ren* Channel. This should be done several times. Next, conduct pushing-massage several times along the same route. Carry out this procedure in cooperation with Head and Face Exercise and Neck Exercise.

If you feel distending pain around the point *Dazhui* (Du 14), you may apply pushing manipulation on *Dazhui* (Du 14) and *Jizhong* (Du 6) and pat downward along the Du Channel several times. This therapeutic method may be used for the treatment of stagnation and blood stasis in any location. Administration of drugs dispersing in nature, treatment by outgoing Qi, and acupuncture is prohibited.

2. Treatment with Outgoing Qi. In accordance with Corresponding Channel Point Selection Theory, select the points in and around the location where stagnation and blood stasis exist. Digitally tap and knead the points and push and stroke along the channel. Use the Flat Palm hand gesture and the manipulative procedures of pushing, pulling and quivering to emit Qi so that channel movement is induced. Outgoing Qi is applied along the channel route to guide and normalize the functional activities of Qi and to dredge the channels.

5.1.3 LEAKING OF GENUINE (VITAL) QI

Symptoms. During or after Qigong practice one may experience the sensation of Qi leaking of from the external genitals, anus, or other points. This leaking may not be controlled by the mind or simple breathing practice. Leaking of genuine Qi may lead to wasting and weakness of the extremities, a pale grayish and dark complexion, vexation, failure of mind concentration, spontaneous perspiration, night sweat, seminal emission, insomnia, and reluctance to speak or move.

1. Self-Treatment with Qigong Exercise. Terminate the Qigong exercises that caused the symptoms. Anus contracting, teeth tapping, and saliva swallowing are among other techniques that can often help alleviate symptoms. Another recourse is to pat the *Ren, Du,* and twelve regular channels along the direction of their course to ensure a smoother flow of Qi. The following herbal prescription may be given to bring Qi back to its origin:

Rhizoma Rehmanniae Praeparada (Shudi)	30 grams
Fructus Corni (Shanyurou)	30 grams
Radix Ginseng (Renshen)	9 grams
Magnetitum (Cishi)	30 grams
Radix Achyranthis Bidentatae (Niuxi)	18 grams
Cortex Cinnamomi (Rougui)	6 grams
Os Draconis Fossilia (Shenglonggu)	30 grams
Concha Ostreae (Shengmuli)	30 grams
Cinnabaris (Zhusha)	1 gram taken following its infusion

The above herbs, except Cinnabaris, which is infused separately, are prepared as one decoction and given by oral administration, 5–10 doses altogether.

2. Treatment with Outgoing Qi. Press and knead the following points: *Shenshu* (U.B. 23), *Mingmen* (Du 4), the *Dantian* and *Guanyuan* (Ren 4). Using the Flat Palm hand gesture along with pushing-locating manipulation, emit Qi towards the point *Mingmen* (Du 4). Then use pushing-guiding manipulation to break through the channels and guide Qi to its origin. If Qi leaks from the external genitals, anus, or *Huiyin* (Ren 1), guide it to flow upward to the Middle *Dantian*. If Qi leaks from the sweat pores, close the pores and guide it to flow back to the Urinary Bladder Channel and the Lung Channel. If Qi leaks from the nasal cavity, treatment with outgoing Qi should focus on dredging the Lung and the *Ren* Channels.

5.1.4 MENTAL DERANGEMENT

Symptoms: During Qigong exercises, a phenomenon of mental derangement (also called being infatuated *(Ru Mo)*), may appear in some practitioners who have regarded the illusion emerging during or after Qigong exercise as true. This condition often leads to mental derangement such as uncommunicative and eccentric disposition, a withered and dull expression, apathy, and trance. Some even lose their confidence of living and want to commit suicide. Others suffer from continuous auditory and visual hallucinations, which are similar to that seen in psychotics. These symptoms are known as the ten devils and are described in *Works of Zhong and Lu's Taoist Doctrine (Zhong Lu Chuan Dao Ji)*. The ten devils include: the devil of six thieves, the devil of animals, the devil of aristocracy, the devil of six passions, the devil of love, the devil of adversity, the devil of saints, the devil of fight, the devil of amusement with women, and the devil of sexuality.

1. **Self-Treatment with Qigong Exercise.** Terminate the Qigong exercises that have caused the symptoms. Turn a deaf ear to the auditory hallucination and a blind eye to the visual hallucination, and pay no heed to any illusion. Allow such illusions to emerge and disappear spontaneously. If the symptoms are severe, go and see a doctor for comprehensive treatment. The following prescription, *Baihe Dihuang Tang*, may be used for treatment:

Bulbus Lihi (Baihe)	30 grams
Radix Rehmanniae (Shengdihuang)	30 grams
Concha Ostreac (Shengmuli)	30 grams
Magnetitum (Cishi)	30 grams
Radix Achyranthis Bidentatae (Niuxi)	15 grams
Radix Polygalae (Yuanzhi)	12 grams
Semen Ziziphi Spinosae (Chaozaoren)	9 grams
Cinnabaris (Zhusha)	1 gram taken following its infusion

These drugs, except Cinnabaris, which is infused separately, are decocted for oral administration.

2. Treatment with Outgoing Qi. Open the points of the Eight Extra Channels in accordance with the theory of point selection called The Eight Methods of Intelligent Turtle *(Ling Gui Ba Fa)* and with the principle of opening the points at a definite time. Press and knead the acupuncture points *Baihui* (Du 20), *Dazhui* (Du 14), *Lingiai* (Du 10), and *Feishu* (U.B. 13). Use Flat Palm or Sword Thrust hand gestures and the pushing-pulling-quivering manipulations to emit Qi and guide it to flow along the channels. Pinch the points *Baihui* (Du 20), *Yintang* (Extra 1), *Shangen*, *Renzhong* (Du 26), *Tinggong* (S.I. 19), *Jiache* (St 6), *Quchi* (L.I. 11), *Hegu* (L.I.4), *Weizhong* (U.B.40), and *Chengshan* (U.B.57). Use the Middle Finger Propping hand gesture and the vibrating method to emit Qi towards the points *Jiuwei* (Ren 15) and *Zhongwan* (Ren 12) for a period of 18 normal respirations. Next, guide Qi to flow along the *Ren* Channel back to *Dantian*.

5.1.5 MANAGEMENT OF TEMPORARY SYMPTOMS EMERGING DURING QIGONG EXERCISE.

Some mild symptoms may emerge during the course of initial practice. These symptoms, usually resulting from incorrect exercise, should not be regarded as deviations and are not difficult to treat. Following, are some common symptoms and their management methods:

Fullness of the Head and Headache. Qigong beginners who have not mastered the practicing methods are often nervous mentally. They may hold their facial muscles too tightly or exert too much mind control. Such situations often cause headaches. Treatment methods include relaxation of the mind and muscles in the head during Qigong practice, Head *Daoyin* Exercise, Psychosomatic Relaxation Exercise, and the exercise of saying "Xu" from the Liver Regulation Exercise.

Choking Sensation in the Chest. This symptom usually stems from breath-holding and breath-prolonging. Massaging the Chest and Saying "He", Massaging the Chest and Saying "Si", Chest Exercise, or concentrating the mind on the point *Zusanli* (St. 36) may relieve this symptom.

Abdominal Distention and Soreness. These two symptoms usually occur in beginners who perform the exercise Abdominal Respiration too strenuously. To alleviate the symptom, pay attention to proper movement of the abdominal muscles, use a reasonable time duration for each exercise session, and practice Abdominal Exercise.

Coldness of the Extremities. This symptom is usually due to excess of *Yin* and deficiency of *Yang* or by incorrect Qigong practice in terms of time, posture, and breathing methods. If the symptom is caused by excess of *Yin* and deficiency of *Yang* and if the methods of the practitioner are correct, the *Yang* Qi will recover gradually and the symptoms will disappear. If the symptom is caused merely by incorrect practice methods, you should make the proper corrections and practice the exercise, Taking Essence From the Sun for supplementation.

5.2 Syncope

Syncope, also called fainting, is a state of temporary loss of consciousness, which is usually caused by temporary cerebral ischemia or temporary cerebral anoxia. Syncope is often caused by mental excitement, fright, severe pain, standing for a long period of time, or standing up suddenly. TCM holds that syncope is caused by a disorder of Qi, by Qi deficiency and collapse, or by failure of lucid *Yang* to rise.

Symptoms. The patient is usually weak, experiencing dizziness, blurred vision, shortness of breath, and sweating, followed by fainting. A pale face, cold limbs, low blood pressure, a fine and rapid pulse, and reduced pupils are also common. Acupuncture or massage applied with too much force and treatment with outgoing Qi, may also cause syncope.

1. **Self-Treatment with Qigong Exercise.** When premonitory symptoms of syncope emerge, the following procedures may be applied. Lay supine with the head slightly lowered. Unbutton the collar, relax the whole body, take a deep breath, and use the mind to guide Qi into the *Dantian*. Use the thumb-nail to press the acupuncture points *Renzhong* (Du 26), *Neiguan* (P 6), and *Hegu* (L.I. 4). Relax the arms at both sides of the body and breathe naturally with the tongue on the palate. Relax the head, neck, upper limbs, chest and abdomen, back and waist, and the lower limbs. Practice Relaxation Exercise three times.

2. **Treatment with Outgoing Qi.** Lie supine. Pinch and knead the points *Baihui* (Du 20), *Renzhong* (Du 26), *Neiguan* (P 6), *Hegu* (L.I. 4), and *Taichong* (Liv 3) to invigorate the vital function, replenish Qi, and restore consciousness. Use the Flat Palm hand gesture and the pushing-pulling manipulation to emit Qi toward the lower, middle, and upper *Dantian* in order to activate the functional activities of Qi. Next, use the Flat Palm gesture and the pushing-leading manipulation to guide Qi to the Lower *Dantian* from *Baihui* (Du 20) down along the *Ren* Channel. Finally, dredge Qi to the lower limbs and feet.

Carry out these procedures 3–7 times. When the above procedures are complete, push and stroke the upper and lower limbs along the Three *Yang* Channels of Hand and the Three *Yang* Channels of Foot, using the pushing-stroking manipulation, 3 times. This may regulate the functional activities of Qi and invigorate Qi flow and blood circulation.

5.3 Common Cold

The common cold, known as URI (upper respiratory infection) refers to inflammation of the respiratory tract caused by viruses or bacteria. The disease often occurs during climate changes or decline of the body resistance. TCM regards the common cold as an invasion of wind-cold, wind-heat, or seasonal pathogenic factors.

Symptoms. Symptoms of the wind-cold are headache, nasal obstruction with watery discharge, sneezing, chilliness, anhidrosis, cough with thin phlegm, soreness of the joints, a thin, white tongue coating, and a superficial, tense pulse. Symptoms of wind-heat type are headache with fever or sweating, dry mouth and sore throat, yellow nasal discharge, yellow sticky phlegm, a thin and yellowish tongue coating, and a rapid, superficial pulse.

1. **Self-Treatment with Qigong Exercise.** Assume a sitting or lying posture. Pinch and knead the acupuncture points *Yintang* (Extra 1), *Taiyang* (Extra 2), *Quchi* (L.I. 11), and *Hegu* (L.I.4) with the thumb. Practice Head and Face Exercise and Nose and Teeth Exercise. Dredging the points *Fengchi* (G.B. 20) and *Tianzhu* (U.B. 10) as described in the Neck Exercise. Finally, dredge the Three *Yang* Channels of the Hand, the Three *Yin* Channels of Hand, the Three *Yang* Channels of the Foot, and the Three *Yin* Channels of the Foot as described in Shoulder Arm Exercise and Exercise of the Lower Limbs.

2. **Treatment with Outgoing Qi.** With the patient sitting, pinch and knead the points *Yintang* (Extra1), *Kangong*, *Quchi* (L.I.11), and *Hegu* (L.I.4) to open up the points and normalize the functional activities of Qi. Use the Flat Palm gesture and pushing-pulling manipulation to emit Qi toward *Yintang* (Extra 1) and *Taiyang* (Extra 2). Use the pulling-guiding manipulation to guide Qi to flow downward along the *Ren* Channel and the Stomach Channel of Foot *Yangming* to both feet. Three to seven repetitions of these techniques will expel wind-cold or wind-heat out from the feet along the channels.

   Press and knead the points *Fengfu* (Du 16), *Dazhui* (Du 14), *Fengmen* (U.B.12), and *Feishu* (U.B.13). Emit Qi toward

Dazhui (Du 14), *Fengmen* (U.B.12), and *Feishu* (U.B.13) using the Flat Palm gesture and the pushing-pulling manipulation. Guide the Qi downward along the Urinary Bladder Channel of Foot *Taiyang* with pulling-guiding manipulation. Stop guiding when the functional activities are balanced). Finally, press and knead *Fengchi* (G.B.20), *Dazhui* (Du 14), *Fengmen* (U.B. 12), *Quchi* (L.I. 11), and *Hegu* (L.I.4), as well as both arms.

5.4 Epigastralgia

According to TCM theory, pain in the epigastrium is the main symptom of epigastralgia and is caused by one of three syndromes: hyperactive liver Qi attacking the stomach, insufficiency of the spleen *Yang*, stagnation of Qi, and stasis of blood. Improper diet, climate change, and mental factors may also give rise to epigastralgia.

Symptoms. When this condition is caused by hyperactive liver Qi attacking the stomach, there will be pain and fullness in the gastric region, vomiting and sour regurgitation which gets worse when excited, a taut pulse, and white, thin tongue fur. When epigastralgia is caused by insufficiency of the spleen *Yang*, pain will be relieved by pressing and warming the affected area, the patient will have a poor appetite, flatulence, watery vomitus and stools, clear urine, aversion to cold, a white, thin tongue fur, and a slow pulse. When epigastralgia is caused by Qi stagnation or blood stasis, there will be localized pain and tenderness in the epigastrium, masses in the abdomen, black stool, reddened tongue, and a taut, hesitant pulse.

1. **Self-Treatment with Qigong Exercise.** Practice Psychosomatic Relaxation Exercise and Inner Health Cultivation Exercise. The method Rubbing *Zhongwan* (Ren 12) Area, saying "Hu" and the manipulation procedures of Dredging the Spleen and Stomach described in Spleen Regulation Exercise may be practiced by patients with hyperactive liver Qi which is attacking the stomach and causing Qi stagnation and blood stasis. Patients with insufficiency of spleen *Yang* should use the technique Taking Yellow Qi to regulate the spleen and Dredging the Spleen and Stomach. As described in Spleen Regulation Exercise, Chest-Hypochondrium Exercise and Abdominal Exercise should also be performed.

2. **Treatment with Outgoing Qi.** The patient should lie supine, breathe evenly, relax, and expel any distractions. When exhaling, guide Qi to flow towards the gastric area where pain exists. Knead the location of *Lanmen* (ileocecal) junction with

the right hand and press the point *Jiuwei* (Ren 15) with the middle finger of the left hand. Using the Flat Palm gesture and vibrating manipulation, emit Qi towards the gastric area for a period of 14 normal respirations. The Middle Finger Propping gesture with vibrating manipulation should then be used to emit Qi towards the points *Zhongwan* (Ren 12) and *Qihai* (Ren 6). Qi emission should last for 14 normal respirations. Then, push, rub, and knead the abdomen in accordance with Pushing the Abdomen to separate *Yin* and *Yang*. Use the Flat Palm gesture and pushing-vibrating manipulation to emit Qi towards the point *Zhongwan* (Ren 12). The emitting hand should be above, not on, the area. Emit Qi for a period of 14 normal respirations. The pushing and leading manipulations should then be used to guide Qi to flow towards the *Dantian* along the *Ren* Channel or to flow downward along the Stomach Channel of Foot *Yangming*. Stop emitting when the functional activities of Qi are balanced.

With the patient lying prostrate, knead the points *Pishu* (U.B.20), *Weishu* (U.B.21), *Ganshu* (U.B.18) as well as the entire Urinary Bladder and the *Du* Channel. Emit outgoing Qi using the vibrating manipulation on the points of *Pishu* (U.B.20) and *Weishu* (U.B.21) for a period of 14 normal respirations. The Flat Palm gesture and the pulling-leading manipulations are used to guide the flow of Qi downward along the Urinary Bladder Channel of Foot *Taiyang*.

5.5 Hiccup

Hiccup, called *Da E Te* (belch), is usually caused by spasm of the diaphragm due to excessive intake of raw, cold, or pungent food. It may also be caused by an adverse rise of stomach Qi, that results from the liver Qi attacking the stomach.

Symptoms: The hiccup is continuous, usually lasting several minutes or hours and then ceasing without treatment in the mild cases. In severe cases, it may last for days and seriously interfere with eating and sleeping. If hiccup occurs at a time when the patient has been sick for some time or in a state of severe illness, it may be a sign of crisis which deserves special attention.

1. **Self-Treatment with Qigong Exercise.** Facing south, assume either the sitting or standing posture. Keep the feet shoulders-width apart, and relax the whole body. Practice reverse abdominal respiration taking deep breaths. During expiration, guide the flow of Qi downward to the *Dantian* and then further to

the acupuncture point *Dadun* (Liv.1) for a period of 3–9 normal respirations. Practice Chest-Hypochondrium Exercise and Massaging the Hypochondrium and saying "Xu" of the Liver Regulation Exercise.

2. **Treatment with Outgoing Qi.** The patient should sit or stand facing south, relax, and breath normally. Pinch *Zhongge* (located at the end of the line between the first two-segments of the middle finger on the thumb side). Press and knead the points *Pishu* (U.B. 20), *Geshu* (U.B. 17), *Tanzhong* (Ren 17), *Zhongfu* (Lu 1), and *Yunmen* (Lu 2).

Using the Flat Palm hand gesture and pushing-pulling-leading manipulation emit Qi towards the point *Tanzhong* (Ren 17) and then guide the Qi down to the lower limbs along the Stomach Channel of Foot *Yangming* which helps regulate the functional activities of Qi. Next, emit Qi towards the points *Pishu* (U.B. 20), *Weishu* (U.B. 21), and *Ganshu* (U.B. 17) on the back, and guide Qi to flow downward along the Urinary Bladder Channel of Foot *Taiyang*. This may normalize the functional activities of Qi.

If the patient's condition has not improved, emit Qi towards the point *Baihui* (Du 20) and guide it to flow to the *Dantian* along the *Ren* Channel, which is known as guiding Qi to its origin. All this is performed using the Flat Palm gesture and pushing-pulling-leading manipulations.

5.6 Diarrhea

Diarrhea refers to frequent defecation and loose or watery stool. Improper diet and exo-pathogenic factors may cause gastrointestinal dysfunction that results in diarrhea. The disease is most prevalent in summer and autumn when dampness and heat, the two most common exo-pathogenic factors, are rampant. Deficiency of the spleen or kidney *Yang* may also cause chronic diarrhea.

Symptoms. Symptoms of diarrhea may (in accordance with its causes and characteristics) be classified into three types: diarrhea due to cold, diarrhea due to heat, and diarrhea at dawn. Patients with diarrhea due to cold generally suffer from intestinal gurgling and abdominal pain, loose stool with undigested food, watery stool, frequent clear urination without thirst, and a deep, slow pulse. This type of diarrhea is mostly caused by cold and spleen deficiency. Characteristics of diarrhea as the result of heat are stinking, yellow, loose stool; burning sensation around the anus; thirst, restlessness; dark urine; frequent urination;

yellowish tongue fur; a wiry, rapid pulse; and usually fever. Diarrhea at dawn is mostly due to weakness of kidney *Yang*, which results in indigestion of food. The patient will usually loosely defecate, every day at dawn at least 2–3 times.

1. **Self-Treatment with Qigong Exercise.** Practice Automatic Qi Circulation Exercise (counterclockwise direction only) supplemented with the Abdominal Exercise. Patients with diarrhea caused by cold and dampness may practice Filth Elimination Exercise, while patients with diarrhea before dawn may practice Taking Essence from the Sun.

2. **Treatment with Outgoing Qi.** Carry out digital point pressing on the acupuncture points *Pishu* (U.B. 20), *Weishu* (U.B. 21), and *Dachangshu* (U.B. 25) to open the back trans- porting points (*Shu* points). With the tip of the middle finger of the right hand, press the point *Lanmen* (ileocecal junction) while pressing the point *Jiuwei* (Ren 15) with the tip of the middle finger of the left hand to help normalize the functional activities of Qi.

Apply the Flat Palm gesture and vibrating manipulation to emit Qi toward the points *Zhongwan* (Ren 12), *Tianshu* (St. 25), *Duqi* (S 35 the umbilicus), and *Guanyuan* (Ren 14) for a period of 14 normal respirations. Massage the abdomen 36 times. The massage will have a tonifyng effect if the case is due to a deficiency syndrome and a purging effect if the case is due to an excess syndrome.

Apply the Flat Palm gesture and pushing-pulling manipula- tion to emit Qi towards the abdomen. Guide the Qi to rotate in a clockwise or counterclockwise direction, then guide it to flow downward along the Stomach Channel. Next, push from the coccyx up to the seventh thoracic vertebra with a flat palm. Then press and knead the Urinary Bladder Channel (both sides) and the point *Zusanli* (St. 36).

For patients with diarrhea at dawn, use the Flat Palm gesture and pushing-rotating manipulation to emit Qi towards *Mingmen* (Du 4, gate of life) and the *Dantian* for a period of 9–10 normal respiration cycles. For patients with diarrhea due to cold and dampness or due to heat and dampness, use the Flat Palm gesture and pulling-guiding manipulation to guide Qi to flow downward along the Stomach Channel. Continue to guide Qi out of the body through the points *Zusanli* (St. 36) and *Jiexi* (St. 41), or through the toes.

5.7 Constipation

Constipation may be regarded as a single disease or as a complication of other diseases. There are six common causes of constipation: deficiency, excess, wind, cold, Qi stagnation, and heat. Deficiency implies a *Yang* or *Yin* deficiency of the lower *Jiao (Xia Jiao)*. If deficiency of *Yang* occurs, *Yin*-Qi may stagnate and fail to circulate. If deficiency of *Yin* occurs, secretion of the body fluid may become imbalanced giving rise to dryness in the intestines. Excess refers to excess syndrome of the stomach, which causes constipation through poor food digestion. Wind implies an unbalanced circulation system, which cannot easily eliminate waste. Cold implies the accumulation of pathogenic cold, which impairs the functional activities of Qi. Qi stagnation implies the energetic impairment of Qi. Heat refers to the heat that hinders the secretion of the body fluid.

Symptoms. Symptoms of constipation are usually dry and hard stool, prolonged duration or infrequency of defecation and difficulty in defecation though the patient has strong desire to defecate. Infrequency of defecation usually means every 3–5 days or even 6–7 days. Clear urine, dry stool, and difficulty in defecation are usually found among patients with constipation due to cold and deficiency. Dark urine and preference for cold food are seen among patients with constipation due to excess and heat. Cough, difficulty in breathing, cold extremities, fullness and distention of the abdomen and difficulty in defecation are found among patients with constipation due to wind and cold. Belching, depression in the chest and abdomen, and fullness and distention in the chest and hypochondrium are found among patients with constipation due to Qi stagnation.

1. **Self-Treatment with Qigong Exercise.** Practice Automatic Qi Circulation Exercise with an emphasis on clockwise turning. Abdominal Exercise may also be used.

   Patients with constipation due to excess, heat, deficiency, or cold should also practice Rubbing *Zhongwan* and "Hu" described in Spleen Regulation Exercise.

2. **Treatment with Outgoing Qi.** Press and knead the points *Dachangshu* (U.B. 25), *Shenshu* (U.B. 23), *Ciliao* (U.B. 32) and the eight-*liao* points (on the sacrum) to induce movement in the back (*Shu*) points. Then, push *Qijiegu*, the seven-segment bone, 50 times.

   Break through the point *Lanmen* (Extra 33) with the thumbs and the middle fingers of both hands. Next, emit Qi using Flat Palm gesture and vibrating manipulation, toward the point *Zhongwan* (Ren 12) for a period of 14 normal respiration cycles. Emit Qi with the Dragon Mouth gesture and pushing-rotating manipulation towards the point *Tianshu* (St. 25) for a period of 14 normal respirations. Continue by emitting Qi, with the same gesture and manipulation, towards the point *Guayuan* (Ren 4) for a period of 8 normal respirations. Guide Qi to rotate clockwise. Emit Qi with the hands above the area to be treated for a period of 8 normal respirations using Flat Palm gesture and pushing-pulling-rotating manipulation, and then guide Qi to rotate clockwise to get its functional activities normalized.

5.8 Hypochondriac Pain

The cause of hypochondriac pain was clearly explained in *The Yellow Emperor's Canon of Internal Medicine (Huang Di Nei Jing)* which says, "Pain occurs below the hypochondrium when pathogenic factors invade the liver." Though hypochondriac pain may also be caused by Qi stagnation, accumulation, channel blockage, phlegm stasis, deficiency and excess, it is always related to the liver and is commonly seen among patients with hyperactivity of liver *Yang* or stagnation of the liver Qi.

Symptoms. Hypochondriac pain on one side is more common than on both sides. Severe pain, cough, and difficulty in breathing are seen among patients with excess syndrome. When patients possess excessive fire in the liver one may see hypochondriac pain on both sides, a taut pulse, and a bitter taste in the mouth. Weak pulse, dry throat, poor appetite, and dull or stinging pain are found among patients with deficiency syndromes, including insufficiency of liver and kidney *Yin*.

1. **Self-Treatment with Qigong Exercise.** Practice of Massaging the Hypochondrium and "Xu" of the Liver Regulation Exercise is beneficial for patients with excess syndrome. Taking Black, which is included in Kidney Regulation Exercise, is beneficial to patients with deficiency syndrome. Chest Hypochondrium Exercise will also help alleviate this condition.

2. **Treatment with Outgoing Qi.** Conduct digital tapping, pressing, and kneading on the points *Tanzhong* (Ren 17), *Qimen* (Liv 14), *Zhangrnen* (Liv 13), *Ganshu* (U.B. 18), *Geshu* (U.B. 17), *Zhigou* (S.J. 6), and *Yanglingquan* (G.B. 34) in order to break through them. This will also promote the flow of Qi and the circulation of blood in the Liver Channel.

   Emit Qi using Flat Palm gesture and pushing-pulling-leading manipulation towards the painful region for a period of 11 or 22 normal respirations. Guide Qi, with pulling-leading manipulation, to flow downward along the Liver Channel. Tap the point *Guanyuan* (Ren 4) and knead the point *Shenshu* (U.B. 23). Emit Qi using the Flat Palm gesture and quivering manipulation toward the lower abdomen, with the point *Guanyuan* (Ren 4) as the center, for a period of 8 or 16 normal respirations.

5.9 Bronchitis

Bronchitis is a disease of the respiratory tract with cough as its main symptom. Acute bronchitis is caused by bacterial or viral infection or by irritation from protracted smoking. Chronic bronchitis is caused by frequent attacks of acute bronchitis or other diseases. TCM holds that bronchitis is classified into cough, cough with dyspnea, and phlegm retention, and is often caused by the pathogenic factors of wind-cold, wind-heat, or excess of phlegm-dampness.

Symptoms. Acute bronchitis is often manifested as cough due to exopathy. The onset is acute with symptoms of infection of the upper respiratory tract such as nasal obstruction, itching throat, and dry cough, accompanied by fear of cold, fever, headache, and general malaise. The cough is paroxysmal, with thin or thick phlegm, the tongue fur is white and thin, and the pulse floating and tense. If pathogenic wind-cold is transmitted into the interior of the body and causing heat syndrome, symptoms and signs such as yellow tongue fur, thick or purulent phlegm, a floating and rapid pulse, or a slippery and rapid pulse will occur.

Chronic bronchitis is usually manifested by cough due to internal injury. The cough is frequent and increases in the fall and winter or during climate changes. The cough will becomes severe early in the morning and at nightfall. The patient may have abundant phlegm and slippery and greasy tongue fur. A slippery pulse indicates excess of phlegm-dampness manifested as abundant expectoration, purulent phlegm, and phlegm with blood. A thin and rapid pulse indicates injury of the collateral branches of the Lung Channel by heat. If attacks of chronic bronchitis are too frequent and the disease lingers, pulmonary emphysema will develop.

1. **Self-Treatment with Qigong Exercise.** If the patient is suffering from deficiency syndrome, practice Taking White Qi of the Lung Regulation Exercise. Practice Rubbing the Chest and "Si" of the Lung Regulation Exercise if the patient is suffering from excess syndrome. Both types of patients should practice "Regulating the Lung and Guiding Qi from the Lung Regulation Exercise as well as Chest-Hypochondrium Exercise.

Patients suffering from acute bronchitis, with the symptoms of an exterior syndrome such as headache and aversion to cold, may practice Nose and Teeth Exercise and Head and Face Exercise.

Those with deficiency of the spleen and lung Qi, may practice Taking Yellow Qi included in the Spleen Regulation Exercise.

Those with deficiency of kidney Qi may practice Taking Black Qi included in the Kidney Regulation Exercise. All of the above patients may practice Health Promotion Exercise.

2. **Treatment with Outgoing Qi.** With the patient sitting, press and knead the points *Tanzhong* (Ren 17) and *Feishu* (U.B.13). If the patient is affected by external pathogenic factors (such as wind and cold), the points, *Kangong*, *Taiyang* (Extra 2), and *Fengmen* (U.B. 12) should be massaged. Using Flat Palm gesture and pushing-pulling-quivering manipulations, emit Qi towards the points *Tanzhong* (Ren 17) and *Feishu* (U.B.13) for a period of 6 or 12 normal respirations. Next, guide the channel Qi to flow along the Lung Channel.

Emit Qi with vibrating manipulation towards the point *Zhongwan* (Ren 12) for a period of 14 normal respirations. Then, with Flat Palm gesture and pushing-leading manipulation, guide Qi to flow downward along the Stomach Channel.

For patients with deficiency of lung or spleen Qi, emit Qi with Flat Palm gesture and pushing-pulling manipulation, towards the points *Zhongwan* (Ren 12) and *Qihai* (Ren 6) for a period of 8 normal respirations, and then guide Qi to flow along the *Ren* Channel to its origin.

If the patient has deficiency of kidney Qi, Flat Palm gesture and pushing-pulling-leading manipulations are used to emit Qi towards the *Dantian* and *Mingmen* (Du 4) for a period of 8 normal respirations.

If the patient has wind-cold syndrome due to exuberant exopathy, Flat Palm gesture and pulling-leading manipulations are applied to emit Qi towards the point *Tanzhong* (Ren 17) and to guide Qi to flow along the Lung Channel and out of the body through the fingertips.

5.10 Bronchial Asthma

Bronchial asthma is an allergic disease usually characterized by repeated attacks and paroxysmal dyspnea with wheeze. TCM holds that this disease is caused by, invasion of wind-cold, improper diet, mental depression, deficiency of the spleen and lung due to fatigue, accumulation of phlegm-dampness in the lung, impairment of the ventilating and dispersing functions of the lung, slipperiness of primordial Qi in the lower part of the body, and failure of the kidneys in receiving lung Qi (deficiency of kidney-Qi may cause dyspnea).

Symptoms. Bronchial asthma falls into two types, excess syndrome and deficiency syndrome. The former is manifested by acute onset dyspnea, which often makes the patient keep his mouth open and shoulders raised to gasp for breath. The patient may also experience fullness in the chest, wheezing, a floating and tense pulse, and thin, white tongue fur. The latter is characterized by shortness and rapidness of breath, severe wheezing upon movement, pale face, sweating, cold extremities, a light-red tongue, and a thin, weak pulse.

1. **Self-Treatment with Qigong Exercise.** Practice Psychosomatic Relaxation Exercise, Inner Health Cultivation Exercise, and Chest-Hypochondrium Exercise. Patients with the excess syndromes of Qi stagnation or phlegm-dampness should also practice Rubbing the Chest and "Si," which is included in the Lung Regulation Exercise. Patients, with deficiency of spleen and lung Qi should also practice Taking White Qi and Taking Yellow Qi which are included in Lung Regulation Exercise and Spleen Regulation Exercise respectively. Patients with failure of the kidneys in receiving Qi or with sweating and shortness of breath should practice Taking Black Qi, which can be found in Kidney Regulation Exercise.

2. **Treatment with Outgoing Qi.** Carry out digital tapping and kneading on the points *Dingchuan* (Extra 17), *Tiantu* (Ren 22), *Tanzhong* (Ren 17), *Guanyuan* (Ren 4), *Feishu* (U.B. 13), *Pishu* (U.B. 20), and *Shenshu* (U.B. 23). Emit Qi using Flat Palm gesture and vibrating manipulation towards *Dingchuan* (Extra17), *Feishu* (U.B. 13), and *Pishu* (U.B. 20) for a period of 14 or 28 normal respirations. With the hands above the body surface, guide Qi with pushing-pulling manipulation to downward along the *Du* Channel to *Mingmen* (Du 4). Guide Qi this way 3–7 times. Using Dragon Mouth or Flat Palm gesture and pushing-pulling-quivering manipulations, emit Qi towards the points *Tiantu* (Extra 17) and *Tanzhong* (Ren 17). Guide Qi to flow along the *Ren* Channel to the *Dantian*, which can make the adversely ascending Qi descend.

   If the patient suffers from kidney deficiency and insufficiency of the kidney *Yang*, the Flat Palm gesture and pushing-pulling manipulations should be used to emit Qi towards the points *Mingmen* (Du 4) and *Shenshu* (U.B .23), and the *Dantian* to strengthen the kidney *Yang*.

If the patient has phlegm accumulation and dampness due to hypo-function of the spleen, press and knead the point *Fenglong* (St. 40). Emit Qi using pulling-leading manipulation towards *Tanzhong* (Ren 17) in order to guide Qi to flow to the Stomach Channel of Foot *Yangming* so that the phlegm can be expelled out of the body along the Stomach Channel and through the point *Zusanli* (St. 36).

5.11 Palpitation

Palpitation refers to the abnormal heartbeat (cardiac impulse) that can be felt by patients. It is a common symptom of neurosis and heart diseases of various kinds. TCM holds that palpitation is actually irritability caused by fright or insufficiency of Qi and blood that fails to nourish the heart.

Symptoms. Palmus is the main symptom, sometimes accompanied by chest distress, nausea, and vomiting. Palpitation is paroxysmal, usually induced by mental irritation, overstrain and excessive drinking or smoking.

1. **Self-Treatment Qigong Exercise.** Practice Health Promotion Exercise, Inner Health Cultivation Exercise, and Chest-Hypochodrium Exercise. Patients with excess syndrome may practice Rubbing the Chest and "Ha" and Regulating the Heart and Guiding Qi, which are included in Heart Regulation Exercise. Patients with deficiency syndrome may practice Taking Red Qi and Regulating the Heart and Guiding Qi described in Heart Regulation Exercise. Patients with insufficiency of kidney Qi may practice Strengthening the Kidney and Guiding Qi found in Kidney Regulation Exercise as a supplement.

2. **Treatment with Outgoing Qi.** Press and knead the points *Xinshu* (U.B. 15), *Ganshu* (U.B. 18), *Tanzhong* (Ren 17), *Jiuwei* (Ren 15), and *Lanmen* (ileocecal junction) to open them and to activate their functional activities of Qi. Apply the Middle Finger Propping or the Sword-Thrust gesture and vibrating manipulation to emit Qi towards each of the points *Xinshu* (U.B. 15), *Ganshu* (U.B.18), and *Tanzhong* (Ren 17) for a period of 8 normal respirations. Then guide the Qi to flow to the *Dantian*.

   Patients with fright or dysphoria may be treated with Dragon Mouth hand gesture and vibrating manipulation and Qi may be emitted toward *Jingming* (U.B. 1), *Yintang* (Extra 1), and *Baihui* (Du 20) for a period of 8 normal respirations each. The doctor may continue to emit Qi with the hands above these points and guide Qi downward using pulling-leading manipulation to ensure a smooth flow of Qi.

5.12 Seminal Emission

There are two main types of seminal emission: nocturnal emission and spermatorrhoea. Nocturnal emission is usually caused by excess of ministerial fire, exuberance of the heart-*Yang*, deficiency of kidney-*Yin*, overstrain, and breakdown of the normal physiological coordination between the heart and the kidney. Spermatorrhoea is caused by failure of the kidney in storing reproductive essence and incompetence of the genitals in discharging seminal fluid.

Symptoms. Nocturnal emission refers to ejaculation when dreaming. It occurs once every 5–6 nights, or every 3–4 nights, and is accompanied by dizziness, vertigo, fatigue, and abdominal pain. Spermatorrhoea refers to ejaculation not related to dreaming. It may occur at any time or upon thinking of sexual activities. Patients with spermatorrhoea often have lassitude of the extremities and poor memory. The disease can last for years.

1. **Self-Treatment with Qigong Exercise.** Waist Exercise, Kidney Regulation Exercise, and Exercise for Nourishing the Kidney for Rejuvenation may be practiced to treat this problem.

2. **Treatment with Outgoing Qi.** Press and knead the acupuncture points *Shenshu* (U.B. 23), *Xinshu* (U.B. 15), *Mingmen* (Du 4), (Ren 4), *Zhongji* (Ren 3), and *Sanyinjiao* (Sp 6). Using Flat Palm gesture and vibrating manipulations, emit Qi towards *Zhongwan* (Ren 12), *Guanyuan* (Ren 4), and *Mingmen* (Du 4) for a period of 8–12 normal respirations. Emit Qi with Flat Palm gesture and pushing-pulling-quivering manipulation, toward the *Dantian* and *Mingmen* (Du 4) in order to guide Qi to flow upwards along the *Du* Channel to the point *Baihui* (Du 20). Continue guiding the Qi to flow forward along the *Ren* Channel to the *Dantian*.

   Finally, emit Qi using Flat Palm gesture and pushing-leading manipulation toward *Baihui* (Du 20) for a period of 8 normal respirations. Guide Qi to flow along the *Ren* Channel to the *Dantian*.

5.13 Impotence

Impotence is a disease manifesting itself as failure of penis erection or softness of the erected penis. It is usually caused by masturbation in adolescence or in sexual life intemperance. Anxiety, which impairs the reproductive essence, depression, and kidney impairment due to fright, may also give rise to impotence.

Symptoms. Failure of normal erection or softness of the erected penis that collapses quickly are the main symptoms. These symptoms may also be accompanied by lassitude in the loins and legs, dizziness, vertigo, listlessness, and weakness of the limbs.

1. **Self-Treatment with Qigong Exercise.** Practice Exercise for Nourishing the Kidney for Rejuvenation and Waist Exercise. Patients with insufficiency of kidney-Qi may also practice Kidney Regulation Exercise. Patients with physical weakness may also practice Inner Health Cultivation Exercise or Health Promotion Exercise. Patients with listlessness may practice Head and Face Exercise as a supplement.

2. **Treatment with Outgoing Qi.** Press and knead the points *Shenshu* (U.B. 23), *Mingmen*, (Du 4) *Guanyuan* (Ren 4), and *Sanyinjiao* (Sp 6). Using Flat Palm and vibrating manipulation, emit Qi towards *Guanyuan* (Ren 4) for 12 normal respirations. Then, with Middle Finger Propping and vibrating manipulation, emit Qi towards the point *Zhongji* (Ren 3) for 12 normal respirations followed by emitting Qi with Flat Palm and pushing-pulling manipulation toward *Mingmen* (Du 4) for 24 normal respirations.

   Emit Qi with Flat Palm and pushing-pulling-rotating-leading manipulation toward *Mingmen* and the *Dantian* for 24 normal respiration and guide Qi to flow counterclockwise.

5.14 Dysmenorrhea

Dysmenorrhea is a disease characterized by lower abdominal pain during menstruation. It is often related to mental stress during the menstrual period, cold invasion, or cold diet. TCM holds that dysmenorrhea is caused by cold invasion, cold diet, anxiety, anger, emotional depression, and insufficiency of Qi and blood. Dysmenorrhea is classified into two types, excess and deficiency.

Symptoms. Patients with dysmenorrhea of excess type have the symptoms of lower abdominal pain prior to menstruation, interior heat, dry mouth, dark, violet menstrual blood, advanced menstrual period, and usually a taut and rapid pulse. Patients with dysmenorrhea of deficiency type have the symptoms of lower abdominal pain after menstruation, which can be alleviated by warming and hand-pressing, scanty and thin menstrual blood, delayed menstruation, aversion to cold, and a fine, slippery pulse.

1. **Self-Treatment with Qigong Exercise.** Practice Nourishing the Kidney for Rejuvenation and Abdominal Exercise and Waist Exercise. For patients with deficiency syndrome may practice Automatic Qi Circulation Exercise emphasizing clockwise Qi rotation among patients with excess syndrome emphasize counterclockwise Qi rotation. Delicate patients with deficiency syndrome may also practice Health Promotion Exercise or Inner Health Cultivation Exercise.

2. **Treatment with Outgoing Qi.** With the fingertips, press and knead the points *Qihai* (Ren 6), *Guanyuan* (Ren 4), *Zhongwan* (Ren 12), and *Shenshu* (U.B. 40) to open them. Emit Qi using Flat Palm or Middle Finger Propping gesture and vibrating manipulation toward *Zhongwan* (Ren 12) and *Guanyuan* (Ren 4). Conduct circular rubbing on the lower abdomen. This has a replenishing effect in cases with deficiency and a purging effect in cases with excess. Follow this motion by pressing and kneading the points *Sanyinjiao* (Sp 6), *Yinlingquan* (Sp 9), and *Taixi* (K 3).

   Emit Qi towards the Lower *Dantian* using Flat Palm gesture and pushing-pulling-rotating manipulation. Guide Qi to whirl round the umbilicus clockwise for cases with deficiency syndrome, and counterclockwise for cases with excess syndrome.

   Finally, using Flat Palm gesture and fixed quivering manipulation, emit Qi towards the *Mingmen* (Du 4), the point *Shenshu* (U.B. 23), and the sacral region. Guide Qi to flow downward along the Urinary Bladder Channel to normalize Qi activities.

5.15 Stiff Neck

Stiff neck refers to the simple, acute stiffness and pain of the neck that causes cervical immobilization. It is often caused by improper sleeping posture, invasion of pathogenic wind-dampness, or obstruction of channels and collaterals.

Symptoms. Stiff neck is usually noticed in the morning when the patient feels pain on one side of the neck. There may be difficulty in turning the head and sometimes radiation of pain to the shoulder and back. Cervical muscles will be in a spasmodic state, local tenderness will be obvious, but no swelling or local heat will be found.

1. **Self-Treatment with Qigong Exercise.** Practice Neck Exercise and Shoulder-Arm Exercise.

2. **Treatment with Outgoing Qi.** Press and knead the point *Tianzhu* (U.B. 10) and the portion of Urinary Bladder Channel on the two sides of the neck. Next, press and knead the points *Fengchi* (G.B. 20), *Fengfu* (Du 16), *Jianzhongshu* (S.I. 15), *Jianwaishu* (S.I. 4), *Quchi* (L.I. 11), and *Hegu* (L.I. 4). This may help open the points and dredge the channels and collaterals.

   Using Flat Palm gesture and pushing-pulling-leading manipulation, emit Qi towards the painful area of the neck. Guide Qi to flow downward along the Urinary Bladder Channel, and also guide Qi to the upper arms along the Small Intestine Channel. This may help dredge the channels and collaterals and regulate the functional activities of Qi. The oblique-pulling method is applied to the neck to help relieve rigidity of the joints and to regulate the muscles.

5.16 Pain in the Waist and Lower Extremities

Pain in the waist and lower extremities is often caused by invasion of wind-coldness and wind-dampness into the channels and collaterals due to sitting or lying on damp ground. Internal injury caused by over-strains, deficiency, weakness of kidney Qi, insufficiency of vital essence, and trauma are also causes of this disorder. It is a syndrome similar to the symptoms of protrusion of intervertebral disc, sciatica and others.

Symptoms. Those with pain in the waist and lower extremities of the wind-cold-damp type, often have the following symptoms: soreness of the waist, difficulty in waist movement, radiation of pain to the legs or feet in severe cases, aggravation of pain in cloudy weather, and local sensation of coldness. Those, with pain in the waist due to kidney deficiency have symptoms of protracted and dull pain, lassitude in the loins and legs, listlessness, and a rapid, fine pulse. Patients with pain in the waist and lower extremities due to trauma, usually have the symptoms of marked tenderness, mild swelling, and radiating pain along the Gallbladder Channel of Foot-*Shaoyang* or the Urinary Bladder Channel of Foot Taiyang.

1. **Self-Treatment with Qigong Exercise.** Practice Waist Exercise and Exercise of the Lower Extremities.

2. **Treatment with Out going Qi.** Press and knead the points *Shenshu* (U.B. 23), *Mingmen* (Du 4), *Yaoyangguan* (Du 3), *Huantiao* (G.B. 30), *Yanglingquan* (G.B. 34), *Weizhong* (U.B. 40), *Chengshan* (U.B. 57), *Kunlun* (U.B. 60), and *Taixi* (K 3) to dredge the Channels and promote the channel Qi to flow.

Emit Qi, with Flat Palm gesture and pushing-pulling-leading manipulation toward the points *Mingmen* (Du 4) and *Shenshu* (U.B. 23), and guide Qi downward along the Urinary Bladder Channel of Foot *Taiyang*. Using Flat Palm gesture and pushing-pulling-leading manipulations, emit Qi towards *Huantiao* (G.B. 30), and guide Qi to flow towards the lower-extremities along the Gall Bladder Channel of Foot-*Shaoyang* to help dredge the channel. Carry out oblique pulling of the waist, palm-patting, and passive movements of waist, hips, and knees to relieve rigidity of the joints, relax muscles and tendons, and promote blood circulation.

5.17 Headache

Headaches are subjective symptoms that can be found in many acute or chronic diseases. TCM holds that headaches can be caused by the following: internal injury or exopathy (i.e. invasion. of exo-pathogenic wind-cold into the vertex and then into the brain via channels), adverse rising of accumulated stomach-heat, insufficiency of Qi and blood, improper preservation of the *reservoir of marrow* (referring to the brain), stagnation of phlegm-dampness, lucid *Yang* failing to rise, or excessive fire of the liver and gallbladder.

The head is the pivot of all the *Yang* channels, collaterals, and channel-Qi. Collateral-Qi and Qi of the viscera all meet in the head. Headaches of various types are named after the routes of channels (i.e., *Yangming* Headache).

Symptoms

Yangming **Headache (Frontal Headache).** Pain in the forehead (the *Yangming* Channel goes to the forehead along the headline), dry thirst, dysphoria with feverish sensation, foul breath, constipation, yellow tongue fur, and a forceful or slippery, rapid pulse.

Shaoyang **Headache (Migraine—Lateral Headache).** Pain in one or both sides of the head (the Shaoyang channel supplies the sides of the head). Sensation of excessive heat in the head and severe pain are the main symptoms. They are often accompanied by conjunctival congestion, hypochondriac pain, bitter taste in the mouth, dry throat, yellow and dry tongue fur, and a taut, rapid pulse.

Taiyang **Headache (Occipital Pain).** Pain in the posterior aspect of the head (the pathway of the Taiyang channel) is the main symptom which is accompanied by fever, aversion to cold, stiffness and pain in the neck and back, thin, white tongue fur, and a floating tense pulse.

Jueyin **Headache (Vertex Pain).** The Channels of Foot *Jueyin* meet at the vertex (top of head). Thus, pain in the vertex is the main symptom, which is accompanied by vertigo, vexation, quick temper, flushed face, bitter taste in mouth, insomnia, reddened tongue with yellow fur, and a taut and rapid or fine and rapid pulse.

1. **Self-Treatment with Qigong Exercise.** Practice Psychosomatic Relaxation Exercise with emphasis placed on relaxation of the channels related to the pain area.

   Yangming headache. Emphasize relaxation of the Stomach Channel of Foot *Yangming* and the Large Intestine Channel of Hand *Yangming*.

   Shaoyang headache. Emphasize relaxation of the Gall Bladder Channel of Foot *Shaoyang* and the *Sanjiao* Channel of Hand *Shaoyang*.

   Taiyang headache. Emphasize relaxation of the Urinary Bladder Channel of Foot *Taiyang* and the Small Intestine Channel of Hand *Taiyang*.

   Jueyin headache. Emphasize relaxation of the Liver Channel of Foot *Jueyin*.

   Also practice Head and Face Exercise for all the above.

2. **Treatment with Outgoing Qi.** Press and knead the following points according to the location of pain.

   Yangming headaches. Press and knead the points *Yintang* (Extra 1), *Touwei* (St 8), *Hegu* (L.I. 4), and *Zusanli* (St 36).

   Shaoyang headaches. Press and knead the points *Taiyang* (Extra 2), *Xuanlu* (G.B. 5), and *Yanglingquan* (G.B. 34).

   Taiyang headaches. Press and knead the points *Fengfu* (Du 16), *Fengchi* (G.B. 20), *Tianzhu* (U.B. 10), *Jianzhongshu* (S.I. 15), *Jianwaishu* (S.I. 14), and *Houxi* (S.I. 3).

   Jueyin headaches. Press and knead the points *Baihui* (Du 20), *Yanglingquan* (G.B. 34), and *Taixi* (K 3).

When the above points have been selected and massaged then emit Qi towards the pain area using the Flat Palm gesture and pushing-pulling-leading manipulation. Guide Qi downward from the head along the channels with pushing-leading manipulation.

To treat pain on one side of the head, first emit Qi towards the pain area to promote the functional activities of Qi. Next, guide Qi to flow to the fingertips along the *San Jiao* Channel of Hand *Shaoyang* with pulling-leading manipulation. Finally, guide Qi downward to the lower extremities along the Gall Bladder Channel of Foot *Shaoyang*, using the same manipulation, to balance the functional activities throughout the body.

Finally, emit Qi toward the lateral sides, the front, and the back of the head using Flat Palm gesture and pushing-pulling-rotating manipulation to normalize the functional activities of Qi.

5.18 Insomnia

According to TCM, failure to fall asleep is the main symptom of Insomnia, which is caused by over-anxiety, impairment of heart and spleen, loss of essence and blood, improper diet, and impairment of the stomach and intestines.

Symptoms. The main symptoms of insomnia are failure to fall into sleep, falling asleep with difficulty, or broken sleep and difficulty in falling asleep again.

Insomnia of the type *Timidity Due to Insufficiency of Qi and Deficiency of Blood of the Heart* has the additional symptoms of palpitation, excess dreaming, tendency to wake or become frightened, vexation, night sweating, red margin of the tongue, and a taut, fine pulse.

Insomnia of the type *Deficiency of Qi and Blood in the Heart and Spleen* has the following additional symptoms: palpitation, amnesia, fatigue, lack of appetite, pale and dry face, thin and whitish tongue fur, and a fine, weak pulse.

Insomnia of the type *Breakdown of the Normal Physiological Coordination between the Heart and the Kidney* has the additional symptoms of dizziness, amnesia, tinnitus, palpitation, soreness in loins and knees, reddened tongue with less coating, and a fine, rapid pulse.

Insomnia of the type *Incoordination Between the Spleen and the Stomach* has the following additional symptoms: fullness and distention in the stomach and abdomen; belching; difficulty in falling asleep; difficulty in moving bowels; yellowish and greasy tongue fur; and a heavy, slippery, and rapid pulse.

1. **Self-Treatment with Qigong Exercise.** Practice Psychosomatic Relaxation Exercise and Head and Face Exercise.

   Patients with insomnia of the *Timidity Due to Insufficiency of Qi and Deficiency of Blood of the Heart* type may also practice Heart Regulation Exercise.

   Patients with insomnia of the *Deficiency of Qi and Blood in the Heart and Spleen* type may practice Heart Regulation Exercise and Spleen Regulation Exercise.

   Patients with insomnia of the *Breakdown of the Normal Physiological Coordination between the Heart and the Kidney* type may practice the Exercise for Ascending and Descending *Yin* and *Yang*, Heart Regulation Exercise, and Kidney Regulation Exercise.

Patients with insomnia of the *Incoordination between the Spleen and the Stomach* type may practice Spleen Regulation Exercise and Automatic Qi Circulation Exercise.

2. **Treatment with Outgoing Qi.** Digitally tap, press, and knead the points *Dazhui* (Du 14), *Baihui* (Du 20), and *Taiyang* (Extra 2). Push and knead the points *Hanyan* (G.B. 4) and *Shuaigu* (G.B. 8) and tap and knead the points *Ganshu* (U.B.18), *Shenshu* (U.B. 23), *Guanyuan* (Ren 4) and *Qihai* (Ren 6). These procedures can open the points and dredge the channels.

Emit Qi using Flat Palm gesture and vibrating manipulation towards the points *Baihui* (Du 20) and *Dazhui* (Du 14) for a period of 8 or 16 normal respirations.

Emit Qi toward *Zhongwan* (Ren 12) and *Guanyuan* (Ren 14) for a period of 8–16 normal respirations. Then, emit Qi (with hands off the point) towards *Baihui* (Du 20) with Flat Palm gesture and pushing-leading manipulation. Guide Qi to the two points of *Yongquan* (K 1) along the Kidney Channel. The patient should also concentrate his mind on *Yongquan* (K 1).

Again, digitally tap and knead *Baihui* (Du 20) and *Taiyang* (Extra 2). Push *Hanyan* (G.B. 4) and *Shuaigu* (G.B. 8) and digitally tap *Baihui* (Du 20) and *Dazhui* (Du 14). Sway the upper extremities.

To treat patients with insomnia of the type *Timidity Due to Insufficiency of Qi* and *Deficiency of Blood of the Heart*, also emit Qi using Middle Finger Propping gesture and vibrating manipulation towards the points *Xinshu* (U.B. 15), *Ganshu* (U.B. 18), and *Juque* (Ren 14) for 14 normal respirations. Guide Qi with Flat Palm gesture and pushing-leading manipulation along the Heart and the Gall Bladder Channel to balance the functional activities of Qi.

To treat patients with insomnia of the type *Breakdown of the Normal Physiological Coordination between the Heart and the Kidney*, also emit Qi with Middle Finger Propping gesture and vibrating manipulation, towards *Shenshu* (U.B. 23) and *Xinshu* (U.B. 15) for a period of 14 normal respirations respectively. With Flat Palm gesture and pushing-leading manipulation, guide Qi along the Heart and Kidney Channel to normalize the functional activities of Qi.

To treat patients with insomnia of the type *Deficiency of Qi and blood in the Heart and Spleen*, emit Qi, with Middle Finger Propping gesture and vibrating manipulation toward the points *Pishu* (U.B.

20) and *Xinshu* (U.B. 15) for a period of 14 normal respirations. Additionally, guide Qi with Flat Palm gesture and pushing-leading manipulation, to flow along the Spleen Channel so that the functional activities of Qi will become normal.

To treat patients with insomnia of the type *Incoordination between the Spleen and the Stomach*, emit Qi using Middle Finger Propping gesture and vibrating manipulation toward the points *Pishu* (U.B. 20) and *Weishu* (U.B. 21) for a period of 14 normal respirations. With Flat Palm gesture and pushing-leading manipulation, guide Qi along the Stomach Channel to normalize the functional activities of Qi.

5.19 Hypertension

Hypertension refers to a state in which blood pressure is often higher than 18.7/12 KPa (140/90 mmHg) at rest. TCM believes that hypertension is caused by the miscommunication of the liver and kidney, excess of *Yin* and *Yang*, or upward movement of phlegm-dampness.

Symptoms. Patients with hypertension of the type *Flaming-up of the Liver Fire* have the following symptoms: headache, fullness of the head; flushed face and eyes; dry mouth; vexation; tendency to get angry; constipation; yellowish tongue fur; and a taut, rapid, and forceful pulse.

Patients with hypertension of the type *Deficiency of the Liver Yin and Kidney Yin* may also have vertigo; tinnitus; lassitude in the loins and leg; palpitation; insomnia; a dark; red tongue; and a taut, thin, and rapid pulse. In addition, symptoms of phlegm-dampness oppressed feeling in the chest, numbness of the extremities, obesity in appearance, and a taught, slippery pulse may sometimes be seen in patients with hypertension of the two types mentioned above.

1. **Self-Treatment with Qigong Exercise.** Practice Psychosomatic Relaxation Exercise, Head and Face Exercise, Neck Exercise, Upper Limb Exercise, and Exercise of the Lower Limbs.

   Patients with hypertension of the type *Flaming-up of the Liver-fire* should also practice Rubbing the Hypochondrium and "Xu" included in the Liver Regulation Exercise.

   Patients with hypertension of the type *Deficiency of Liver Yin and Kidney Yin* should also practice Kidney Regulation Exercise and Liver Regulation Exercise.

2. **Treatment with Outgoing Qi.** Press and knead the points *Lanmen* (ileocecal junction), *Zhongwan* (Ren 12), and *Guanyuan*

(Ren 4). Push *Tianmen* (life pass), *Kangong* and *Taiyang* (Extra 2). Digitally tap and knead *Pishu* (U.B. 20), *Weishu* (U.B. 21), *Ganshu* (U.B.18), *Danshu* (U.B. 19), and *Zusanli* (St 36). Knead the Urinary Bladder Channel of both sides.

Emit Qi, using Flat Palm gesture and vibrating manipulation toward the points *Baihui* (Du 20), *Dazhui* (Du 14), *Mingmen* (Du 4), *Zhongwan* (Ren 12), and *Guanyuan* (Ren 4) for a period of 8 or 16 normal respirations. Emit Qi with vibrating manipulation toward the point *Zhongwan* (Ren 12) for a period of 8 normal respirations. Emit Qi with Flat Palm gesture and pushing-pulling-quivering- leading manipulations (hand off of the treated parts) toward the point *Baihui* (Du 20) and the *Dantian*. Guide Qi with pushing-pulling-leading manipulation to flow along the lower aspect of the Stomach Channel to balance Qi in the upper and lower parts of the body. Then, guide Qi, with the same manipulation, to flow to the extremities along the Large Intestine Channel of Hand *Yangming* until the functional activities of Qi are normalized.

To treat patients with hypertension of the type *Flaming-up of the Liver-fire*, the Flat Palm gesture and pushing-pulling-rotating manipulation should be applied to emit Qi toward the points *Ganshu* (U.B. 18) and *Shenshu* (U.B. 23) and the *Dantian*.

To treat patients with hypertension of the type *Deficiency of Liver-Yin and Kidney-yin*, Flat Palm hand gesture and vibrating manipulation should be used to emit Qi toward the point *Shenshu* (U.B. 23) and the *Dantian*, which will help nourish the *Yin* of both the liver and kidney.

Diagrams of Acupressure Points

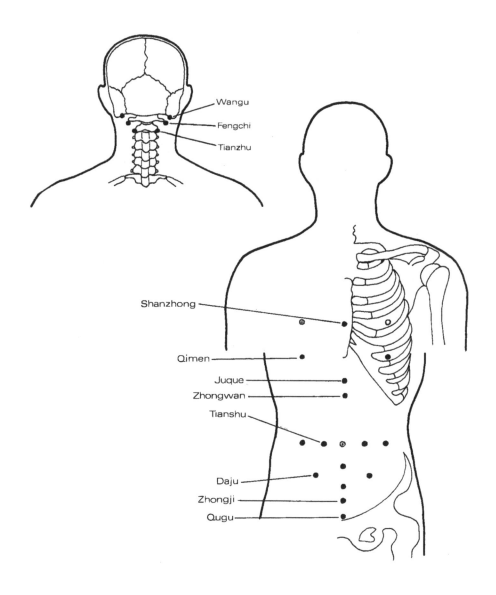

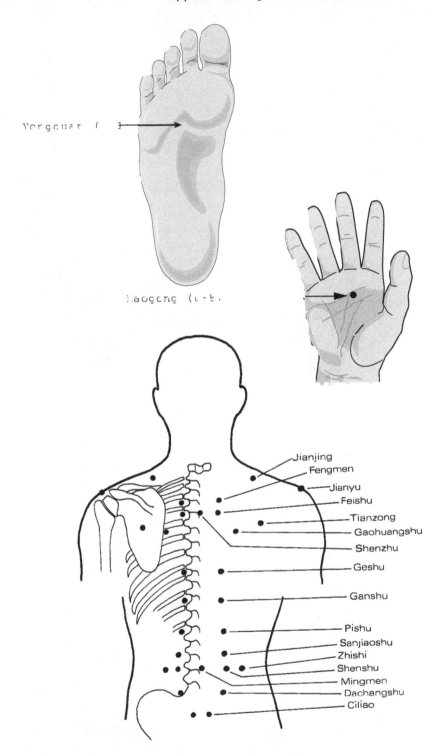

Yongquan (   )

Laogong (   )

Jianjing
Fengmen
Jianyu
Feishu
Tianzong
Gaohuangshu
Shenzhu
Geshu
Ganshu
Pishu
Sanjiaoshu
Zhishi
Shenshu
Mingmen
Dachangshu
Ciliao

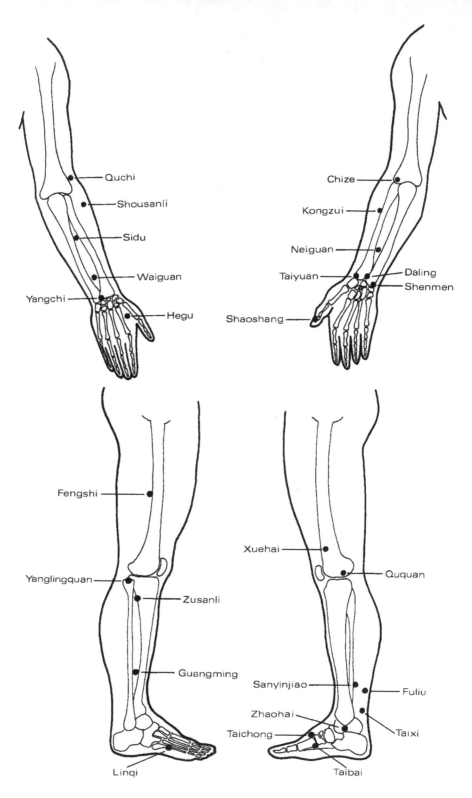

Quchi

Shousanli

Sidu

Waiguan

Yangchi

Hegu

Chize

Kongzui

Neiguan

Taiyuan

Daling

Shenmen

Shaoshang

Fengshi

Yanglingquan

Zusanli

Guangming

Linqi

Xuehai

Ququan

Sanyinjiao

Fuliu

Zhaohai

Taichong

Taixi

Taibai

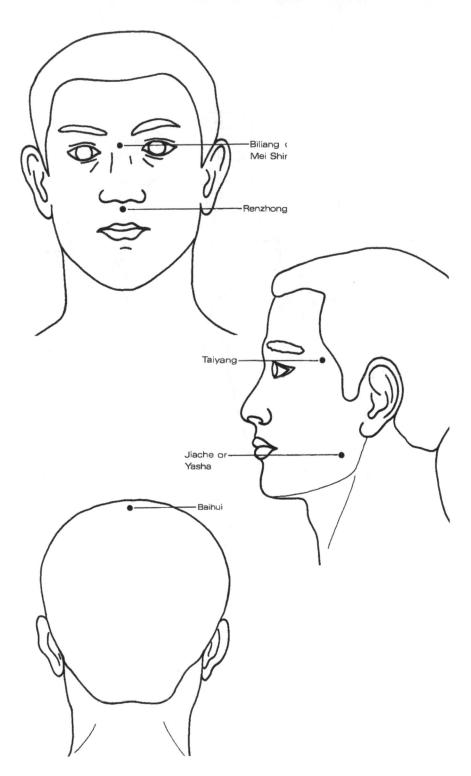

Biliang ‹
Mei Shir

Renzhong

Taiyang

Jiache or
Yasha

Baihui

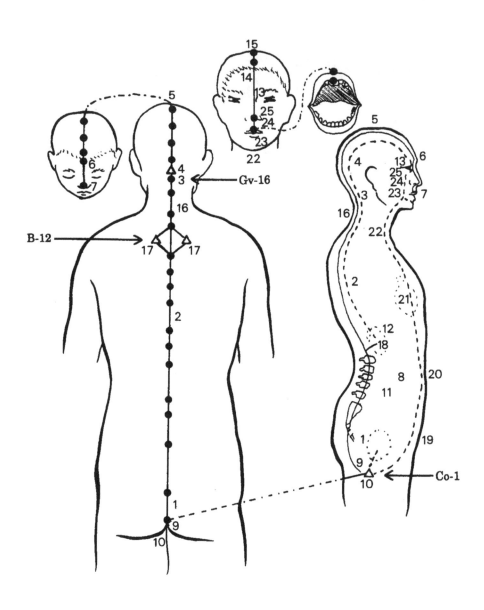

The Governing Vessel (Du Mai)

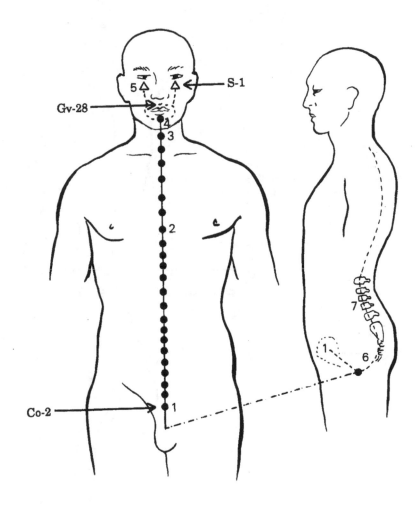

The Conception Vessel (Ren Mai)

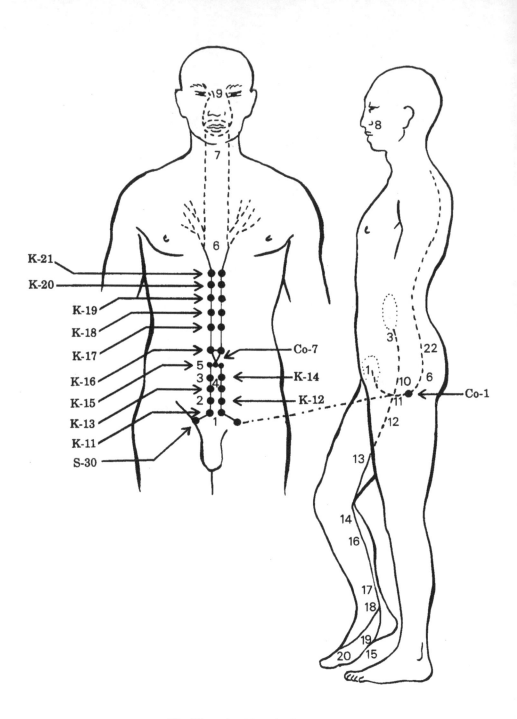

The Thrusting Vessel (Ching Mai)

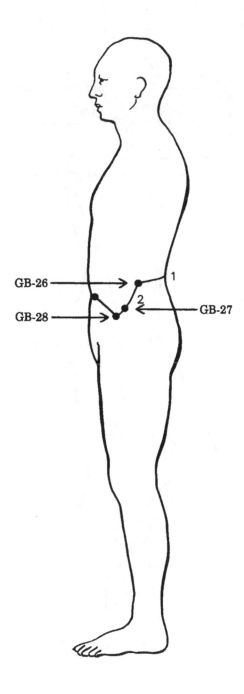

GB-26

GB-28

1

2

GB-27

The Girdle Vessel (Dai Mai)

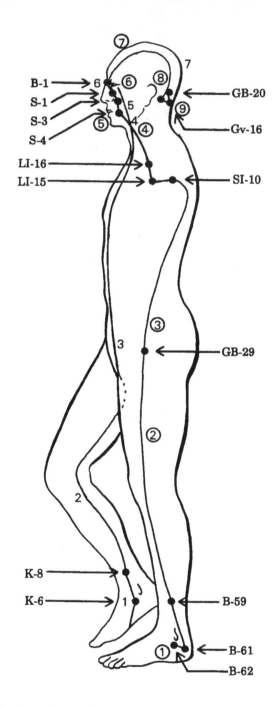

The Yang Heel Vessel (Yangchiao Mai) and the Yin Heel Vessel (Yinchiao Mai)

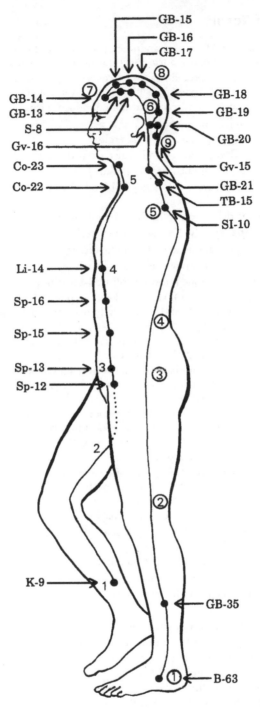

The Yang Linking Vessel (Yangwei Mai) and the Yin Linking Vessel (Yinwei Mai)

Glossary of Terms

Abdominal Breathing Also called abdominal respiration. During respiration the abdomen expands naturally during inspiration and contracts during exhalation

Active Exercise A series of procedures used to expel distracting thoughts, regulate respiration, attain proper posture, and relax both mind and body.

Auricles That portion of the external ear not contained within the head.

Bichi Gong Nose and Teeth Exercise.

Buwei Daoyin Gong Regional Daoyin Exercise.

Cai Rijing Yuehua Gong Taking the Essence from the Sun and the Moon.

Cai-Qi The breathing technique known as taking-in.

Cerebral ischemia Temporary deficiency of blood supply due to obstruction of circulation in the cerebral region.

Cerebral Anoxia Without oxygen in the cerebral region.

Cervical Spondylopathy Any disorder of the vertebrae.

Chang-Xi Breathing technique known as long-breathing.

Chi-Xi Breathing technique known as lasted-breathing.

Chong-Xi Breathing technique known as blurted-breathing

Collaterals Pathways in which Qi and blood are circulated in the human body. Collaterals run transversely and superficially from the meridians.

Da Zhou Tian Large circulation. Literally "Grand Cycle Heaven" after a practitioner completes small circulation, he or she will circulate Qi through his entire body or exchange Qi with nature.

Dantian Locations in the body that are able to store and generate Qi. The Upper, Middle, and Lower Dantian are located, respectively, between the eyebrows, at the solar plexus, and a few inches below the navel.

Daoyin also called Daoyin Massage. A comprehensive exercise that combines specific body posture, breath regulation, and mind concentration with self-massage to develop both the physical and energetic aspects of the body.

Dihui Gong Filth Elimination Exercise.

Directive Mind Concentration The type of concentration that occurs when the flow of Qi is sensed when the mind goes with the movement of the hands or with internal movements of the channels.

Dysmenorrhea Pain associated with menstruation.

Dysphoria an exaggerated feeling of depression and unrest without apparent cause.

Dyspnea Difficulty in breathing sometimes accompanied by pain.

Enteritis Inflamation of the intestines.

Epigastralgia Pain in the pit of the stomach.

Er Gong Ear Exercise.

Essence The most refined part of anything.

Exopathy Pertaining to a disease originating outside the body.

Expectoration The process of spitting out saliva or coughing up materials from the air passageways leading to the lungs.

Fa Gong The emission of Qi.

Fansong Gong Psychomatic Relaxation Exercise.

Fubu Gong Abdominal Exercise.

Fu Lun Zi Zhuan Automatic Circulation Exercise.

Fu Qi Inhalation.

Gastritis Inflamation of the stomach.

Hypertension A condition in which the patient has a blood pressure higher than that judged to be normal.

Hypochondrium Part of the abdomen beneath the lower ribs on each side of the epigastrium.

Jainhi Gong Shoulder Arm Exercise.

Jian Jue Qi emission hand gesture known as Sword Thrust.

Jin-Qi Breathing method known as entering.

Jingxiang Gong Neck Exercise.

Li Wuzang Gong Five Viscera Regulation Exercise.

Liao Fa Shi Jian The practice of qigong therapy.

Lifei Gong Lung Regulation Exercise.

Ligan Gong Liver Regulation Exercise.

Lipi Gong Spleen Regulation Exercise.

Lishen Gong Kidney Regulation Exercise.

Lixin Gong Heart Regulation Exercise.

Long Xian Shi Qi emission hand gesture known as Dragon Mouth.

Lower Jiao Lower portion of the body cavity.

Meridians Pathways in which Qi and blood are circulated in the human body. The meridians, which constitute the main trunks, run longitudinally and within the interior of the body.

Ming Tian Gu A method found in the Ear Exercise called Striking the Heavenly Drum.

Mun-Xi Breathing technique known as full breathing.

Myopia Defect in vision also known as nearsightedness.

Ne Jyang Gong Inner health cultivation exercise.

Ping Zhang Shi Qi emission gesture known as Flat Palm.

Posturization The act of adjusting ones posture before the start of Qigong exercise.

Qi The general definition of Qi is: universal energy, including heat, light, and electromagnetic energy. A narrower definition refers to the energy circulating in animal or human bodies. A current popular model is that the Qi circulating in the human body is bioelectric in nature.

Qiangzhuang Gong Health Promotion Exercise.

Qigong Study, research, and /or practices related to Qi.

Rythmical Mind Concentration That type of concentration that focuses the mind on repetition.

Spermatorrhea Abnormally frequent, involuntary loss of sperm without orgasm.

Shang-Xi Breathing technique known as upper breathing.

Shen-Xi Breathing technique known as deep breathing.

Shengjiang Yin Yang Daoyin Gong Daoyin Exercise for Ascending and Descending Yin and Yang.

Shi-Qi Breathing technique known as eating.

Shugan Mingmu Gong Exercise for Soothing the Liver and Improving Acuity of Vision.

Suggestive Mind Concentration Type of concentration technique that coordinates thought, movement, and language.

Syncope A transient loss of consciousness due to inadequate blood flow to the brain.

Tan Zhua Shi Qi emission hand gesture known as spreading claw.

Thenar Eminence The prominence located at the base of the thumb.

Tinnitus A subjective ringing in the ears.

Tong Ren Du Daoyin Gong Daoyin Exercise for Dredging the Ren and Du Channels.

Toumain Gong Head and Face Exercise.

Wai Qi The emission of Qi.

Xiao Zhou Tian Small Circulation. Literally "Small Heavenly Cycle." In Qigong, when you can use your mind to lead Qi through the Conception and Governing Vessels you have completed Small Circulation.

Xiazhi Gong Exercise of the Lower Limbs.

Xing Ting Automatic Circulation Exercise.

Xiongxie Gong Chest Hypondrium Exercise.

Xiphoid Process The lowest portion of the sternum.

Yan Gong Eye Exercise.

Yangqi Gong Qi Nourishing Exercise.

Yangshen Huichun Gong Exercise for Nourishing the Kidney for Rejuvenation.

Yaobu Gong Waist Exercise.

Zhoutian Gong Circulation Exercise.

Index

Index

BOOKS FROM YMAA

ADVANCING IN TAE KWON DO	B072X
ANALYSIS OF SHAOLIN CHIN NA 2ND ED	B0002
ANCIENT CHINESE WEAPONS	B671
ART OF HOJO UNDO	B1361
BAGUAZHANG 2ND ED.	B1132
CARDIO KICKBOXING ELITE	B922
CHIN NA IN GROUND FIGHTING	B663
CHINESE FAST WRESTLING	B493
CHINESE TUI NA MASSAGE	B043
CHOJUN	B2535
COMPREHENSIVE APPLICATIONS OF SHAOLIN CHIN NA	B36X
CUTTING SEASON—A XENON PEARL MARTIAL ARTS THRILLER	B1309
DESHI—A CONNOR BURKE MARTIAL ARTS THRILLER	E2481
DIRTY GROUND	B2115
DUKKHA, THE SUFFERING—AN EYE FOR AN EYE	B2269
EIGHT SIMPLE QIGONG EXERCISES FOR HEALTH, 2ND ED.	B523
ESSENCE OF SHAOLIN WHITE CRANE	B353
ESSENCE OF TAIJI QIGONG, 2ND ED.	B639
FACING VIOLENCE	B2139
FIGHTING ARTS	B213
FORCE DECISIONS—A CITIZENS GUIDE	B2436
INSIDE TAI CHI	B108
KAGE—THE SHADOW A CONNOR BURKE MARTIAL ARTS THRILLER	B2108
KATA AND THE TRANSMISSION OF KNOWLEDGE	B0266
KRAV MAGA—WEAPON DEFENSES	B2405
LITTLE BLACK BOOK OF VIOLENCE	B1293
MARTIAL ARTS ATHLETE	B655
MARTIAL ARTS INSTRUCTION	B024X
MARTIAL WAY AND ITS VIRTUES	B698
MASK OF THE KING	B114
MEDITATIONS ON VIOLENCE	B1187
MUGAI RYU	B183
NATURAL HEALING WITH QIGONG	B0010
NORTHERN SHAOLIN SWORD, 2ND ED.	B85X
OKINAWA'S COMPLETE KARATE SYSTEM—ISSHIN RYU	B914
POWER BODY	B760
PRINCIPLES OF TRADITIONAL CHINESE MEDICINE	B99X
QIGONG FOR HEALTH & MARTIAL ARTS 2ND ED.	B574
QIGONG FOR LIVING	B116
QIGONG FOR TREATING COMMON AILMENTS	B701
QIGONG MASSAGE	B0487
QIGONG MEDITATION—EMBRYONIC BREATHING	B736
QIGONG MEDITATION—SMALL CIRCULATION	B0673
QIGONG, THE SECRET OF YOUTH—DA MO'S CLASSICS	B841
QUIET TEACHER—A XENON PEARL MARTIAL ARTS THRILLER	B1262
RAVEN'S WARRIOR	B2580
ROOT OF CHINESE QIGONG, 2ND ED.	B507
SCALING FORCE	B2504
SENSEI—A CONNOR BURKE MARTIAL ARTS THRILLER	E2474
SHIHAN TE—THE BUNKAI OF KATA	B884
SHIN GI TAI—KARATE TRAINING FOR BODY, MIND, AND SPIRIT	B2177
SIMPLE CHINESE MEDICINE	B1248
SUNRISE TAI CHI	B0838
SURVIVING ARMED ASSAULTS	B0711
TAE KWON DO—THE KOREAN MARTIAL ART	B0869
TAEKWONDO BLACK BELT POOMSAE	B1286
TAEKWONDO—ANCIENT WISDOM FOR THE MODERN WARRIOR	B930
TAEKWONDO—DEFENSES AGAINST WEAPONS	B2276
TAEKWONDO—SPIRIT AND PRACTICE	B221
TAI CHI BALL QIGONG—FOR HEALTH AND MARTIAL ARTS	B1996
TAI CHI BOOK	B647
TAI CHI CHUAN—24 & 48 POSTURES	B337
TAI CHI CHUAN CLASSICAL YANG STYLE (REVISED EDITION)	B2009
TAI CHI CHUAN MARTIAL APPLICATIONS, 2ND ED.	B442
TAI CHI CONNECTIONS	B0320
TAI CHI DYNAMICS	B1163
TAI CHI SECRETS OF THE ANCIENT MASTERS	B71X
TAI CHI SECRETS OF THE WU & LI STYLES	B981
TAI CHI SECRETS OF THE YANG STYLE	B094
TAI CHI THEORY & MARTIAL POWER, 2ND ED.	B434
TAI CHI WALKING	B23X
TAIJI CHIN NA	B378
TAIJI SWORD—CLASSICAL YANG STYLE	B744
TAIJIQUAN THEORY OF DR. YANG, JWING-MING	B432
TRADITIONAL CHINESE HEALTH SECRETS	B892

more products available from . . .

YMAA Publication Center, Inc. 楊氏東方文化出版中心

1-800-669-8892 • info@ymaa.com • www.ymaa.com

BOOKS FROM YMAA (continued)

TRADITIONAL TAEKWONDO	B0665
WAY OF KATA	B0584
WAY OF KENDO AND KENJITSU	B0029
WAY OF SANCHIN KATA	B0845
WAY TO BLACK BELT	B0852
WESTERN HERBS FOR MARTIAL ARTISTS	B1972
WILD GOOSE QIGONG	B787
WOMAN'S QIGONG GUIDE	B833
XINGYIQUAN, 2ND ED.	B416

DVDS FROM YMAA

ADVANCED PRACTICAL CHIN NA IN-DEPTH	D1224
ANALYSIS OF SHAOLIN CHIN NA	D0231
BAGUAZHANG—EMEI BAGUAZHANG	D0649
CHEN STYLE TAIJIQUAN	D0819
CHIN NA IN-DEPTH COURSES 1—4	D602
CHIN NA IN-DEPTH COURSES 5—8	D610
CHIN NA IN-DEPTH COURSES 9—12	D629
EIGHT SIMPLE QIGONG EXERCISES FOR HEALTH	D0037
ESSENCE OF TAIJI QIGONG	D0215
FACING VIOLENCE—7 THINGS A MARTIAL ARTIST MUST KNOW	D2283
FIVE ANIMAL SPORTS	D1106
KNIFE DEFENSE—TRADITIONAL TECHNIQUES AGAINST A DAGGER	D1156
KUNG FU BODY CONDITIONING 1	D2085
KUNG FU BODY CONDITIONING 2	D2290
KUNG FU FOR KIDS	D1880
LOGIC OF VIOLENCE	D2351
NORTHERN SHAOLIN SWORD —SAN CAI JIAN, KUN WU JIAN, QI MEN JIAN	D1194
QIGONG FOR HEALING	D2320
QIGONG FOR LONGEVITY	D2092
QIGONG FOR WOMEN	D2566
SABER FUNDAMENTAL TRAINING	D1088
SHAOLIN KUNG FU FUNDAMENTAL TRAINING—COURSES 1 & 2	D0436
SHAOLIN LONG FIST KUNG FU—BASIC SEQUENCES	D661
SHAOLIN LONG FIST KUNG FU—INTERMEDIATE SEQUENCES	D1071
SHAOLIN LONG FIST KUNG FU—ADVANCED SEQUENCES 1	D2061
SHAOLIN LONG FIST KUNG FU—ADVANCED SEQUENCES 2	D2313
SHAOLIN SABER—BASIC SEQUENCES	D0616
SHAOLIN STAFF—BASIC SEQUENCES	D0920
SHAOLIN WHITE CRANE GONG FU BASIC TRAINING—COURSES 1 & 2	D599
SHAOLIN WHITE CRANE GONG FU BASIC TRAINING—COURSES 3 & 4	D0784
SHUAI JIAO—KUNG FU WRESTLING	D1149
SIMPLE QIGONG EXERCISES FOR ARTHRITIS RELIEF	D0890
SIMPLE QIGONG EXERCISES FOR BACK PAIN RELIEF	D0883
SIMPLIFIED TAI CHI CHUAN—24 & 48 POSTURES	D0630
SUNRISE TAI CHI	D0274
SUNSET TAI CHI	D0760
SWORD—FUNDAMENTAL TRAINING	D1095
TAI CHI BALL QIGONG—COURSES 1 & 2	D0517
TAI CHI BALL QIGONG—COURSES 3 & 4	D0777
TAI CHI CHUAN CLASSICAL YANG STYLE	D645
TAI CHI CONNECTIONS	D0444
TAI CHI ENERGY PATTERNS	D0525
TAI CHI FIGHTING SET	D0509
TAI CHI PUSHING HANDS—COURSES 1 & 2	D0495
TAI CHI PUSHING HANDS —COURSES 3 & 4	D0681
TAI CHI SWORD—CLASSICAL YANG STYLE	D0452
TAIJI & SHAOLIN STAFF—FUNDAMENTAL TRAINING	D0906
TAIJI CHIN NA IN-DEPTH	D0463
TAIJI 37 POSTURES MARTIAL APPLICATIONS	D1057
TAIJI SABER CLASSICAL YANG STYLE	D1026
TAIJI WRESTLING	D1064
UNDERSTANDING QIGONG 1—WHAT IS QI? • HUMAN QI CIRCULATORY SYSTEM	D069X
UNDERSTANDING QIGONG 2—KEY POINTS • QIGONG BREATHING	D0418
UNDERSTANDING QIGONG 3—EMBRYONIC BREATHING	D0555
UNDERSTANDING QIGONG 4—FOUR SEASONS QIGONG	D0562
UNDERSTANDING QIGONG 5—SMALL CIRCULATION	D0753
UNDERSTANDING QIGONG 6—MARTIAL QIGONG BREATHING	D0913
WHITE CRANE HARD & SOFT QIGONG	D637
WUDANG KUNG FU—FUNDAMENTAL TRAINING	D1316
WUDANG SWORD	D1903
WUDANG TAIJIQUAN	D1217
XINGYIQUAN	D1200
YANG TAI CHI FOR BEGINNERS	D2306
YMAA 25 YEAR ANNIVERSARY DVD	D0708

more products available from . . .

YMAA Publication Center, Inc. 楊氏東方文化出版中心

1-800-669-8892 • info@ymaa.com • www.ymaa.com

Printed in the USA
CPSIA information can be obtained
at www.ICGtesting.com
JSHW082213140824
68134JS00014B/596

9 781886 969704